SHAPE YOUR LIFE:
BODY AND MIND

SHAPE YOUR LIFE: BODY AND MIND

S.Chitrai Kani

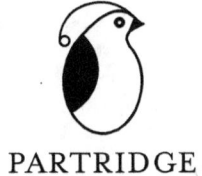

PARTRIDGE

To order additional copies of this book, contact
Partridge India
000 800 10062 62
orders.india@partridgepublishing.com

www.partridgepublishing.com/india

CONTENTS

With fond memories of

my mother Karuppayi alias Punka Maram
my uncle P. Theriappan
my brother S.Sakkarai

my teachers

Mr Natarajan
Class VII-B, Kaleeswari Middle
School, Vanniyampatti, and
Mr Prince,
Class IX-A, CMS High School, Srivilliputtur,

who shaped my life and influenced my thoughts.

INTRODUCTION

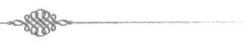

This book is meant for those who are in their twenties, but it may take many years to understand even though all the topics were discussed, argued, and fought for and against from the beginning of the evolution of human beings.

Those who live a comfortable life and perfectionists who see life in 'black or white' or 'yes or no' or 'good or bad' may take more time to understand this book. They need a lot of experience in life to understand what life is.

But life being so complex, with each one having a different experience and different impact in mind, what one says about life may not be fully agreeable to another, what is agreeable may not be fully done, what is done may not be fully satisfactory to others, etc. Even those who are placed in the same situation may feel differently.

There is nothing new in this book. Only old thoughts told by common man and the wise are presented *briefly* without any special jargon. The topics covered have been discussed and interpreted in many ways for centuries by all - from common man to great thinkers and philosophers - depending on the needs and experiences of the evolving society.

Experience in life transcends different faiths, religions, castes, and complexions, the rich and the poor, etc. even though these attributes are also a part of their experiences. Each one undergoes the same experience of pleasure and pain in different times and places, but depending on the level of selfishness and perception of past experiences, life is shaped in the mind uniquely.

As the great astrophysicist Stephen Hawking thought, the mistakes in the creation of the universe brought varieties of materials on earth. Similarly, the mistakes done by the humans and the surrounding environment have brought out a unique life to each one with a different understanding or different perceptions and thoughts.

So anyone not agreeing with the opinion of the author has an absolute right to disagree. But an introspection or review after new experiences in life may help to narrow down the level of disagreement, if not fully agreeing with the author. But in life, sane words are rarely heard in time; even if heard, they are rarely followed. Those who are conditioned from childhood on unquestioned faiths and beliefs or illogical customs and rituals may find certain views blasphemous or sinful unless they see the world.

Life flows along with the struggle for survival within the society and against other societies inimical to one's own society. Figuratively speaking, neither a deer can hide itself always from a tiger, nor can a tiger hunt down a deer whenever it pleases. Life is delicately balanced within the society.

Some points in some topics may be repeated in some other topics since many aspects of life are interrelated.

With micro-families, social life and sharing experiences are minimized nowadays. Hope, this book will help all to think in spite of isolated social lives and busy schedules in life.

To avoid duplication of the title of the book, the title of the 2014 publication is slightly modified. The topics are rearranged based on health, physio-psychological, metaphysics, etc. for selective reading at any time. The first 50% of the book can be read from the beginning. The last 25% of the topics may be appreciated more by those who are in their 50s and 60s and those who have enough experience in life. Most of the topics are independent and prefer to read topics of your interest selectively.

S. Chitrai Kani

FOOD

i) The food that we take is a nutrient for growth and maintenance of our body when taken in right quantity and in right time.

ii) It is a medicine when different kinds of food is taken in right quantity and in right time.

iii) Any kind of food is a poison when taken in excessive quantity at any time.

Just like any machine has a capacity, our stomach and other digestive organs like liver, pancreas, etc. have limited capacity in handling specific nutrients in food like sugar, fat, etc. *at any time*. Hence, too much intake of a specific food at any time may lead to overworking by some parts of the body. Any overworked part may develop fatigue, or it may collapse later. So, overeating food, particularly *rich* food, spoils our health.

Rich foods have too much nutrients of a particular kind, like meat, oil, sugar, etc. Enriched foods are those rich foods which are made more rich by adding different rich foods, like milk sweets, fried meat, etc. or by processing the same rich food, like cheese, milk powder, etc.

For proper digestion of food, our stomach needs water for digestion and space for flexible compression. So leave enough space for water while eating.

Our stomach needs more blood supply for digesting food. So avoid heavy physical work immediately after taking a stomachful of food. Heavy work may cause diversion of more blood to other parts of our body like hands, legs etc.

For proper health, our body needs a variety of nutrients which are available in different types of food even though the primary needs are carbohydrates, proteins and fats which are needed for the growth and maintenance of our body and for doing any work. No single cereal, millet, pulse, vegetable, or fruit is endowed with all the nutrients in right quantities. So prefer to eat a variety of food, particularly seasonal vegetables, greens, and seasonal fruits.

A good food, when overeaten, is harmful to the body, creating uneasiness, flatulence, loose motion, vomiting, and other associated problems. Also, the part of the body which processes the food may malfunction due to overload, or the part of the body that utilizes that nutrient in the food may not be in a position to utilize that much food.

Different chemicals in the food help repair the damaged parts of the body and fight against diseases. They are also needed for the creation and working of different components of our immune system. So the food that we eat is a medicine when eaten in limited quantities, and the same is turned into a harmful thing like poison when overeaten, for they may harm certain parts of our body.

With essential reserve stored for future emergency use, as long as the food that is eaten is utilized completely to do necessary physical and mental work, our body remains healthy.

FOOD AND VARIETY

Each food is unique in its nutrients. What is in a small gooseberry may not be in an apple, and even if it is, it may not be in the right quantity. Since our body needs a variety of nutrients and since no single food is rich in all nutrients and since different parts of the body process or need different types of nutrients, it is better to eat a variety of food, particularly all types of vegetables and seasonal fruits.

Our body is a very big chemical factory, and different parts of our body secrete or use different chemicals for the proper functioning of our body. Tears, saliva, sweat, urine, phlegm, blood, different types of digestive juices, etc. need different chemicals. There are innumerable good bacteria which process different types of food in the intestines and prepare different chemicals for our body. Which food contains all these chemicals?

To put it differently, our hair, skin, nails, teeth, tongue, etc. are made of different materials. Our heart, lungs, stomach, liver, kidneys, blood, bones, etc. are made of different materials. From which food are all those parts of our body made up? Of course, we do not know. Since no food is rich in all nutrients which are needed for different parts of our body, prefer to eat a variety of food for a healthy body. We do not know which food is needed for which part of the body and in which quantity. So, the food should include all types of vegetables, seasonal fruits, greens, and if possible, different types of millets and pulses.

Many internal organs produce or use a lot of chemicals and communicate with related organs through electrochemical messages. Chemicals like insulin, if eaten, are destroyed in the stomach. But all those chemicals should be produced in the body itself in time, when needed, from the food we eat. So prefer to eat a variety of food (and not selective food).

Women not taking a variety of food including different kinds of vegetables, greens, and seasonal fruits are likely to suffer infertility related problems including white discharge.

FOOD AND EATING

What a person eats is for growth, health and for doing productive work. Also, the food affects the mind. Some types of food, like liquor, may give instant energy which may kindle one to do something which is inconceivable. Also, the feeling of shortage of food or abundance of food affects one's mind and shapes one's behaviour and outlook towards life.

While hungry, avoid eating a few morsels of food like a bite of chocolate since it will cause to secrete more acid in the stomach, and in the long run, it may cause ulcer in the stomach. When hungry, at least a quarter stomachful of food should be taken with more water.

Water is a food which helps digestion. Not drinking sufficient water will lead to constipation and uncontrolled flatulence. Some of the water is absorbed by the body directly from the stomach. Drinking water on an empty stomach is not advisable unless one feels very thirsty since it may affect the secretion of acid in the stomach and its flow to the intestines. Sometimes if taken too much on an empty stomach, it may lead to the common cold or wet blocked nose.

Also, our stomach needs some space for the smooth contraction and expansion of the stomach. So overeating will affect proper digestion.

Rich foods[1] like oily food, sweets, meat, liquor, cheese products, etc. need more water for proper digestion. So eat a little less if the food is very rich.

It is better to avoid overeating rather than suffer the consequences. It is more harmful to eat only food of a particular kind (for example, only sweets or meat or oily food and the like) since it will give more stress to one type of organ which processes that particular kind of food even though all parts of the digestive system are involved.

Mix food with saliva while eating so that it helps in the digestion. Bite small amounts of food and chew the food well in the mouth while eating. It will help digestion. Avoid eating mouthfuls of food in a hurried way, for it may choke the throat, and it may not be possible to breathe. In that case, drink a little water *immediately*. To avoid choking, prefer to drink a mouthful of water before you start eating.

Always take medicines after taking food unless advised by a doctor otherwise. Taking medicines in an empty stomach may cause ulcers.

Medicines contain many chemicals, and our food pipe (oesophagus) is sensitive to most of the chemicals. So always drink water after taking medicines. That will clean the chemicals attached to the food pipe.

The medicines that one is taking may create long-term or short-term side effects. Our food contains different chemicals which may react with strong chemicals in medicines producing unwanted and harmful by products. Take medicines in right quantity and in right time, as advised by the doctor.

---

[1]   Rich foods are rich in nutrients. For example, milk boiled for a long time is rich. Milk powder is highly enriched.

Too much refined food or enriched food without roughage may create constipation and other associated problems like colon cancer. So prefer natural food or simple cooked food on most of the days which gives a sense of *fullness in the stomach*.

Each food is endowed with nutrition or minerals in specific combinations by nature. So prefer to eat a variety of food, including seasonal fruits and vegetables. Being choosy in eating may lead to long-term and short-term health problems. Of course, nutrition breeds a big industry.

Never do any hard work like playing, fast cycling, riding on rough roads, etc. immediately after taking food. Gas problems in the intestines may arise since the blood supply needed for the digestion of the food would be diverted to the legs, hands, etc. If one has to do heavy work after meals, prefer to eat half stomachful of food.

Spices like ginger, pepper, etc. have medicinal value. Eat them along with food and in small quantities. Avoid taking them in an empty stomach.

Before taking breakfast, prefer to go to the toilet and pass the stool so that the solid and gaseous wastes in the intestines are removed. That will help to avoid stomach ache or uneasiness or skin-related diseases. Also, before taking stomachful of food as in lunch or dinner, go to toilet so that the related muscles are relaxed and the trapped gas in the intestines is released as flatulence.

Avoid taking milk or tea, or coffee, with milk on a full stomach since milk will take more time to digest and more gas will be produced. Also, avoid taking milk after vomiting or loose motion. Children digest milk fully. But, as one grows more and more, milk is digested less and less.

Our body needs water for digesting the food, maintaining body temperature, taking essential nutrients to body tissues, and removing the waste produced by the body. So drink sufficient quantity of water to purify the blood by the kidneys and the skin. Lack of sufficient water in the blood may damage the kidneys, or stones may be formed, particularly after taking rich food including non-vegetarian food, medicine, alcohol, etc. Let water be the last food taken after eating meals, breakfast, etc.

Just like our brain and heart refresh themselves by reducing their workload during sleep, reduce the workload of the digestive system by skipping a lunch once in a week, fortnight, or in a month, particularly if you are habituated to eat in time without feeling hungry.

FOOD AND NUTRIENTS

The major requirement of our body is carbohydrates for maintaining our body and for doing any work. Starchy foods like wheat, rice, corn, millets, potato, etc. as well as sugar and alcohol are rich in Carbohydrates. Starchy foods will be digested slowly. Sugar will be digested quickly. Alcohol will be digested more quickly and it will be absorbed into the blood directly from the stomach. Too much sugar will strain the pancreas and kidneys, if taken more at a time. Processed carbohydrates will be stored in the liver in the form of glycogen. Eating more starchy foods give a sensation of fullness in the stomach. Sugar may be taken in very limited quality and alcohol may be avoided unless one needs instant energy.

Protein is needed for growth and for repairing our body tissues. Small children need more protein for their growth. It is rich in pulses, meat, fish, egg, etc. Protein is needed in small amounts and it will take more time to digest. Excess protein, if not used by our body, is excreted by the kidneys.

Fat is needed in small amounts. Fat is also an energy-giving nutrient which is rich in edible oil and animal fat. Fat will take more time to digest. Eating more fat at a time may strain the liver and gall bladder. Fat can be stored in the body.

Our body needs vitamins and minerals in very small quantities to prevent diseases and for proper health.

Vitamins A, D, E, and K are *fat-soluble*, and they can be stored in the body. Not taking sufficient fat with our food may affect the absorption of fat-soluble Vitamins. Vitamins B and C are *water-soluble*, and excess amount is removed by the kidneys except some parts of vitamin B which are removed through the faeces. So vitamins B and C should be consumed regularly.

Vitamin A is good for the skin and eyes. It is rich in carrots, broccoli, sweet potato, milk, butter, cheese, egg yolk, liver, etc.

Vitamin B or B complex refers to eight different chemicals and helps in different functions in the body. It is, particularly, very useful for the nervous system. It is rich in animal organs (liver, kidneys, heart), eggs, green leafy vegetables, whole grains, nuts, milk, mushrooms, etc.

Vitamin C is good for the gums. It is an antioxidant which helps in neutralizing the tissue-damaging effects of free radicals which are highly reactive. It is rich in fresh fruits, particularly citrus fruits, pineapple, guava, and berries. It is also rich in fresh vegetables like cabbage, broccoli, tomato, etc. Ancient seafarers used sprouts of some millets to get Vitamin C. Vitamin C gets spoiled if it is over cooked or boiled.

Vitamin D is produced by our body with the help of sunlight. Lack of vitamin D may cause skeletal deformation. Around 30 minutes exposure daily to the sun is good. Be physically active under the sun to avoid sun burn. Water in the perspiration will absorb the skin-damaging ultra-violet rays and heat from the sun.

Vitamin E, which plays some role in red blood cell formation, is rich in vegetable oils, liver, and green leafy vegetables.

Vitamin K, which is essential for blood coagulation, is rich in egg yolk, liver, and green leafy vegetables.

There are many more benefits due to vitamins. Overeating vitamins is also not good for health.

Minerals are chemicals needed by our body in minute quantities like compounds of calcium, phosphorus, potassium, iron, zinc, etc. Their deficiencies can be avoided by eating a variety of food including different kinds of millets, pulses, milk, vegetables, seasonal fruits, green leafy vegetables, etc.

Water is not a nutrient but helps a lot in maintaining body temperature, carrying the nutrients to the body tissues, and in removing the body waste from the body. Not drinking sufficient water may cause dehydration and the formation of stones in the kidneys.

Which nutrients are to be eaten and by how much? Eat more of starchy foods which give a sense of fullness in the stomach with less of sugary foods, less of meat, less of fat or oil and, each day, prefer to take a different kind of seasonal vegetable, greens or a seasonal fruit. In case, you take stomachful of enriched food like fried chicken, cheese, milk sweets, etc. occasionally, skip the next meal and drink more water.

Normally, a little extra food or a little shortage will not affect the body functions. Sometimes, our body tries to adjust its functioning with available food – perennial, excess, or perennial shortage, of nutrients – and that is the beginning of problems for our body including diseases, damage to some parts of our body or cells, deficiency diseases, etc. So prefer to eat a balanced food daily, that is, a variety of food.

FOOD AND OVEREATING

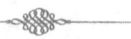

The requirement of different nutrients for our body might have forced the instinct of a child to overeat when a different cuisine is brought and the stomach is full. But overeating by a grown-up is not desirable.

If the bowel movement is not smooth, it may be due to overeating in the previous day. In that case, drink more water and eat after a few hours. If there is problem even after that, then skip the next meal.

Due to overeating, undigested food enters the intestines, which creates gas problems and constipation. If the waste gas is not released as flatulence, the gas may create stomach pain. In that case, go to toilet *and then* drink a glass of water. That may help to relax the muscles in the anus and release the gas as flatulence and relieve pain. If necessary, attend to the call of nature and excrete the solid waste from the body, which will help avoid skin diseases.

In case the waste gas accumulates too much, it will mix with blood and dampen the mood besides causing pimple-like or corn-type protrusions on the skin. Neat habits and medicines may not be able to cure the pimple-type swellings permanently unless the root cause of pimples—that is, overeating—is stopped. Gas in the blood may affect the joints, particularly the knees. Constipation and gas problems may also cause skin diseases.

Waste in our body, if it mixes with blood, is a poison for our body. Constipation and gas trouble makes the body absorb the solid waste and waste gas in our blood which shocks the internal organs and adversely affects their smooth functioning.

When one overeats, the body processes more nutrients and hence produces more chemical wastes (chemical salts like urea). If the chemical wastes are not removed from the blood by the kidneys or the skin, our internal organs may be stupefied and they may work in a stressful environment which may cause hypertension.

Sometimes, overeating causes vomiting and diarrhoea, creating unpleasant conditions besides the long-term effect of obesity. If the body absorbs all nutrients due to overeating, then it causes obesity.

Diarrhoea depletes the minerals and nutrients besides sending out good bacteria from the intestines that help our body process food. In that case, in a glass of pure water, add a spoonful of sugar and a pinch of common salt and drink so as to replenish the lost water. Then, consult a doctor. For some time, avoid eating food, particularly milk, since the bad bacteria may find a medium to thrive. Milk also takes more time to digest and more gas is produced while processing it which may cause vomiting.

Just like sugar or fat, there is no place to store excess protein in our body. Overeating food like meat, chicken, fish, etc. may damage the kidneys in the long run, if more water is not taken with food, since the excess protein is excreted by the kidneys.

Overeating sweets may cause diabetes which, in turn, may damage the kidneys and eyes besides causing high blood pressure and heart failure.

Overeating fatty foods, particularly animal fats, may cause heart failure in the long run besides overloading the liver.

Overeating salty foods may increase blood pressure which, in turn, may affect the kidneys and hence other organs like the heart, eyes, nerves, etc.

Drinking too much liquor may cause diabetes. It may also cause liver cirrhosis, in the long run. Certain foods like meat, milk, etc., if taken without adequate water, may produce stones in the kidneys.

Taking excessive medicines may damage the kidneys since unwanted chemicals are normally removed by the kidneys. Simple tablets used to relieve body pain and fever may damage the kidneys if taken excessively *at any time*. Commonly available tablets that help to reduce body pain and prevent heart attack by its anti-clotting properties of blood may cause stomach ulcer in the long run.

Eating a stomachful of refined or enriched food may result in constipation, and in the long run, it may cause colon cancer.

Overeating general food makes the belly bulge which, in turn, affects the expansion of the lungs. That affects breathing and hence affects the body's metabolism as a whole. So after eating food and drinking water, the stomach level should be almost along the chest level.

Overeating vitamins also has side effects affecting the body.

Not eating sufficient quantities of nutrients also affects the body. So prefer to eat a balanced food- a variety of food, particularly different types of vegetables and seasonal fruits. Avoid being choosy in eating, particularly one or two types of food like sweets or fatty foods and the like.

FOOD AND BEHAVIOUR

The food one takes is used for physical and psychological needs. The behaviour of a person can change depending on the assured availability or scarcity of food and the type of food one takes.

Since food is a periodical requirement, the assured availability of balanced food in the right time has a good psychological effect and creates confidence in the mind. Rising food price was one of the important causes for the French Revolution.

The psychological impact of food on one's mood is tremendous. The effect of liquor on both the body and mind is not always good. A hungry soldier is ready to surrender to an enemy rather than opposing or killing him. So the ancients preferred to feed the guests and relatives both on festivities and death in the name of elaborate rituals.

Unless the food that is eaten is utilized for the betterment of both the body and the mind in the form of work, the stagnant effect of food on both the body and the mind will be immense. That is, what we eat should come out in the form of work and energy, to avoid diseases.

Festivities are associated with enriched food and happiness. Festivals are celebrated on a few days in a year. With abundance of food and affordability, if one wants to celebrate with rich and enriched food frequently, our body may not cope with the workload and some parts of our body may collapse very soon. On most of the days, eat a variety of simple food including vegetables and seasonal fruits which gives a sense of fullness in the stomach.

LIQUOR

Liquor is a food relished by humans from time immemorial. It gives instant energy for a tired person besides sedating the mind.

Liquor, just like any enriched food, should be taken in a limited quantity. If taken in excess, it is good neither for the body nor for the mind. The *'excess'* feeling will not be felt since too much sugar is embedded in a small amount of liquor and the stomach will never have the feeling of *'fullness'* even if the body receives more than the required sugar.

For those who work hard physically, liquor is a food and tonic if taken in a limited quantity. If taken in excess, it is a poison which may spoil the body and mind.

Liquor is a sedative and affects that part of brain which coordinates body movements. So it is one of the major causes of accidents in highways, and hence, it is better to avoid it before driving any vehicle. That is, our body and mind does not work in coordination, if liquor is taken in excess.

Also, the toxic effect of liquor on the functioning of liver is known. Avoid taking liquor on empty stomach.

As a food, liquor needs a lot of water for digestion. Without adequate water, the chance for the formation of kidney stones is more.

Even though people know the ill effects of drinking, why do people get themselves drunk? When a small quantity of liquor can boost the morale and bring out a sense of well-being, why not a little bit more? That little irresistible extra liquor brings out enormous effects affecting the body.

OBESITY

Obesity is not a disease, but it is the cause of many diseases indirectly.

Our body tries to save nutrients from energy-giving food like starchy food (carbohydrates), sugar, or oily food (fat) for future use. But when the stored energy is not used for work by the body and the storage facility exceeds the limit coupled with the intake of more protein (meat, beef, etc.), our body becomes obese. If you eat more, then work more to avoid obesity.

Sometimes, our body has its own mechanism when we overeat food—either we vomit or there is loose motion.

Obesity starts from infants. Overzealous parents feed the infants with more and more enriched food and tonics which causes the infants to lose the sensation of *fullness* in the stomach. Overfeeding by parents may be to fatten the child or to avoid feeding the child in short intervals of time.

To avoid obesity, eat simple balanced food and feel the fullness in the stomach. To feel the fullness in the stomach after eating, most of the food should be simple starchy food (like simple food prepared from wheat, rice, corn, roots, millets, etc.) with less amount of rich foods like oily food, fish and meat products (protein), sugar, and still less amounts of vitamins and minerals which are present in various types of food including whole grains, pulses, vegetables, fruits, and green leafy vegetables. Leave enough space for water which is essential for digestion. Enriched food like fried meat, milk powder, cheese, milk sweets, alcohol, etc. should be kept to a minimum.

After eating and after drinking water, one should feel the *fullness* in the stomach. With a full stomach, the level of the belly should be approximately the level of one's chest. On the next day, one should not have constipation or gas problems associated with flatulence. Overeating will lead to a pot belly, and it will affect the expansion of the lungs. That will affect the breathing which will affect the body's metabolism. That, in turn, will burn less sugar and fat.

Eating a stomachful of simple food is not the same as eating a stomachful of enriched food where more nutrients are to be processed. A stomachful of enriched food will lead to constipation and flatulence problems on the next day. Furthermore, it will lead to more storage of sugar and fat on different parts of the body, straining themselves to process the excess nutrients eaten by us, and at the same time, give stress to kidneys which remove the excess nutrients and the waste produced.

Eat well and work well to avoid obesity. Play or do some physical work or exercise to dissipate the excess energy stored in the body. More and more storage of fat may cause obesity. When hungry, avoid eating a few morsel of food which may kindle more hunger. Avoid sitting for more than one hour continuously. Walk or do some work standing for about 15 minutes every hour.

Eating is a diversionary work for idle persons. So keep yourself busy with some work or hobby. Reading books, singing a song, drawing pictures, using some musical instruments, doing household work, going on tour, etc. will make one busy.

Avoid eating while doing any work. Eating snacks while watching television, reading a book, etc. will make one crave for more unintentionally. While feeling hungry, give yourself some time and eat stomachful of simple food. Avoid eating intermittently.

Even obese persons need all types of nutrients. So, obese people can eat a variety of simple food, including a variety of vegetables and seasonal fruits. They can skip a meal or fast for a day in a week. They can also drink a glass of water before meals to fill the stomach. They should avoid weight-reducing diets which are not balanced in nutrients. Once overweight, avoid reducing the weight overnight which will affect the normal functioning of the body. The weight reduction should be slow and steady. Play with friends or do useful physical work like going to market.

Our body is controlled and managed by different chemicals produced by different parts of our body. Deficiency or oversupply of chemicals may affect the body metabolism and hence the body size. So to avoid obesity, eat a variety of food including vegetables and seasonal fruits so as to get different minerals and produce different chemicals in our body. Also, most of the food should be simple with more roughage which would give a satisfactory feeling of fullness, and at the same time, a considerable part of the food is sent out by our digestive system as waste later. Ensure that what you eat comes out in the form of useful work for good health and to avoid obesity.

DISEASES

If Eve's curiosity to eat the forbidden apple landed Adam and Eve in this world, it was the curiosity of Pandora to see what was in the forbidden Pandora's box[2] that spread all kinds of diseases, vices, and sorrows. Leaving aside such popular beliefs, let us try to find the causes of diseases.

Of course, balanced food, personal hygiene, and a neat environment help to avoid many diseases. Lack of essential vitamins and nutrients cause diseases and malfunctions in the body.

There are innumerable bacteria, viruses, fungi, microbes, etc. in the air, water, food, etc. that will find a suitable person to reside in where they can multiply that it is quite impossible to protect oneself from all kinds of diseases. Besides that—leaving aside mosquitoes, flies, etc. which are carriers of diseases—we have poison in the polluted air and water and contaminated or spoiled food which may cause serious health problems. That is, the environment outside our body is hostile and incomprehensible. So, keep your body fit to fight the diseases by providing different chemicals by eating

---

[2] In Greek mythology, Pandora was the first woman on earth created by the god Hephaestus. She was sent to earth with many gifts, including a box which should not be opened. She opened it out of curiosity, and all types of diseases and sorrows came out of the box.

a variety of food, including all types of vegetables and seasonal fruits every month.

Our body is an integration of different systems, with each part of the system doing some specific work. The different systems of our body, like the respiratory system, digestive system, nervous system, etc. do different works for our body. Even though each part of the body does its work independently, its effect is felt by the different parts of other systems in the body. That is, each part of the body or each system integrated in the body is interdependent. For example, lungs absorb pure air(oxygen), but the heart circulates to the body, and all parts of the different systems, including heart, stomach, kidneys, lungs, brain, etc., which depend on the pure air for working properly.

The food or chemical needed for maintaining, or for proper functioning of, each part, or system, of the body is different and in varying quantities. Fat that soothes the skin and gives energy to our body may cause heart attack; the dust that soothes the soles of our feet may harm the eyes; the common salt that kills some of the bacteria in the mouth and throat may cause blood pressure; the sugar that gives energy to our body may cause diabetes; the lime juice that may prevent some diseases may damage the tooth enamel; the sunlight that creates vitamin D for body may cause cataract in the eyes; etc. That is, there is no unique food which is needed for the whole of our body nor is there a panacea for all ills since the requirement of each part of our body is different.

Broadly speaking, bacteria and viruses cause diseases. The factors that affect diseases are genetics, food and chemicals, physical work, and the environment.

Food may have a major impact on diseases including the genetic factors since food is also a medicine. So prefer to eat a variety of food, particularly seasonal fruits and vegetables. Each food, small or big, makes its own impact on certain parts of the body. *Never think that only costly food has more nutrients.* A cheap berry may be our body's requirement.

A variety of food keeps the body healthy and hence keeps the diseases away. So do not be choosy in eating. The human inclination towards sweets, fatty foods, liquor, and meat are known. Eat everything in limited quantities to avoid diseases.

To cure one disease, do not bring another disease. That is, an overdose of any medicine to cure a disease may bring its own side effects later. *Most of the serious diseases occurring at a young age are due to medicinal side effects or due to overdose of medicines.*

Prefer to inhale pure air and to drink clean water to avoid diseases, and as a responsible member of the society, try to help to maintain the environment neat and clean.

Keep your body neat and clean by taking bath daily or, if the climate is very cold, frequently in a week.

Exercises and physical activities help maintain the body properly by supplying essential nutrients to all tissues and by removing wastes produced by them. Prefer useful physical work and games compared to exercises.

Always tell all the symptoms of the disease to the doctors so that they can diagnose the disease properly and in time. Prefer a doctor who tries to diagnose your disease with the help of symptoms and with minimal dependence on machines and advises how to prevent the disease in future. Keep in mind that health-care is a big business and is no more a noble profession.

Different bacteria prefer different places like the skin, tooth, gums, lungs, intestines, etc. to grow and settle, and they need different chemicals to be killed. There is no universal medicine or antibiotic to kill all these bacteria. So avoid self-medication and consult a doctor before taking medicines. If the right antibiotic medicine is not taken in right quantity in right time during the course of treatment, the bacteria may develop resistance to the antibiotic medicine and it is very difficult to kill the bacteria with that medicine.

In the intestines, there are innumerable good bacteria processing our food and producing different chemicals needed for our body. One of them converts milk into curd! If we take antibiotics orally for any disease, it may kill all bacteria including the good bacteria in the intestines. It may cause loose motion within a few days.

Our body has a mechanism to repair the damaged parts or fight the diseases. We can help by providing proper food and clean air and, if necessary, medicines to our body. But we cannot replace our body's mechanism with medicines. Viruses have to be killed or removed by our body, and medicines cannot do that work. Of course, we can prevent some virus infections by vaccinations.

Sometimes, symptoms are cured and the disease causing the symptoms is not cured, resulting in the repeated occurrence of symptoms or lifelong medications. What doctors cannot cure, you have to cure yourself. Try to find out what food increases or decreases the disease, what kind of work aggravates the disease, what type of environment you were in, what kind of symptoms it produced, etc., and then consult the doctor with details.

SYMPTOMS AND DIAGNOSIS

Different parts of our body give enough distress signals when in trouble. It is up to us to recognize them and take necessary corrective steps for a healthy life. Unless we observe the symptoms correctly and tell them, doctors may find it difficult to diagnose the disease correctly.

Fever is a symptom commonly noticed by all, mostly due to the common cold. The lungs will be infected, and the colour of the mucus may become greenish, or it may smell foul.

Periodic fever (fever coming at a specific time each day) or intermittent fever, may indicate serious diseases like typhoid or malaria or some other diseases which may need blood tests to diagnose.

Fever, cough, or any persistent symptom like pain for more than six days may indicate some serious problem in the body which may need the doctor's attention immediately.

Yellowish urine may indicate an infection of the urinary tract or the kidneys, in which case we have to drink more water to wash the bacteria down the urinary tract. (Vitamin B tablets also cause yellowish urine which is normal). Yellowish-orange or yellowish-brown urine may indicate dehydration of our body, and we have to drink more water. Paining sensation at the end of urination may indicate the formation of kidney stones.

Even after drinking more water, yellowish urine may indicate jaundice. Also, the eyes will become yellowish after a few days. Take simple food and take rest. Consult a doctor.

Stool with a foul smell or greenish colour may indicate an infection in the intestines. (When we take food like green leafy vegetables, the stool may become greenish which is normal.) If black stool comes almost daily, it may indicate internal bleeding of the intestines. (Sometimes when we eat food rich in iron, the stool may become blackish which is normal.) Stool tinted with blood or oozing-out blood along with the stool may indicate piles. Avoid sitting for a long time. Walk or run frequently each day.

Repeated headaches, particularly after taking a bath may indicate sinusitis. Dry the hair immediately after taking a bath and do not apply oil before the hair becomes dry. Headaches after reading books may indicate an eye defect, or the book is not read keeping in the right distance (at least one foot away from eyes - If there is more light, it should be kept still farther). An irritating noise may cause headache, particularly for those without enough sleep. Improper breathing, particularly fast exhalation may cause headache. While standing, take deep breath towards the forehead, keep it for about five seconds in the lungs, and then exhale slowly.

A pain in the ear may be due to less pressure inside the ear which, in turn, may be related to the common cold or infection in the throat or nose. Inhale more air, and closing your nose and mouth, pump air into the nose for immediate relief. Consult a doctor, if the pain persists. Sometimes, it may be due to infected throat and the pain in the ear can be reduced by gargling* with warm salt-water.

Rapid deterioration of eyesight or blurred vision may be due to glaucoma which needs the immediate attention of doctors. Reading books by keeping it closely (less than 1foot) or playing mobile games by keeping it closely may cause eye defect, called short-sight or myopia.

A sudden appearance of pimples or corn-type swellings may indicate serious gas trouble in the stomach or intestines. Overeating leads to gas trouble and constipation. Go to toilet, then drink a glass of water and then excrete solid waste, preferably before breakfast. While standing, take deep breath towards the forehead, keep it for about five seconds and exhale slowly to avoid constipation. This breathing exercise may be done for about 15 minutes in the morning and evening daily.

Skin diseases may be related to constipation and gas trouble (flatulence) which, in turn, may be related to overeating or not drinking sufficient water. Remove body wastes in time.

Stomach pain after taking food may indicate gas trouble or constipation. Take food after going to the toilet. Pain in the stomach when hungry may indicate ulcer. Eat food in time.

A small light-coloured patch or lesion in the skin without sensual feeling to touch may indicate infection of leprosy. Consult a doctor immediately.

While coughing, if sputum is laced with blood, it may indicate tuberculosis. Consult a doctor immediately.

Swelling legs or a shiny calf may indicate sitting for long hours or some other problems related to the internal organs. Walk or do some physical work by standing or moving frequently.

Blocked nose or infection in the throat may cause some pain in the chest sometimes. If one inhales a lot of air and keeps it for a few seconds in the lungs and then exhales slowly, but instead of beating in a fast pace, if the heart beats irregularly (palpitation) or if there is a sense of pain in the heart, then there is some problem in the heart. Consult a doctor immediately.

A discharge from the nipple when the breast is massaged gently or a lump in the breast may indicate breast cancer. Consult a doctor immediately.

An itching skin may indicate lack of oil in the skin. An itching or tender mole in the skin or black spots under the nails may indicate skin cancer. Be active, and avoid sitting, under the sun.

If there is back pain, it may be due to a thick mattress or due to sleeping in the wrong posture or due to a sudden starting or stopping of vehicles.

If there is neck pain or stiff neck, it may be due to the following habits:

i) a thick pillow while laying down in the bed.
ii) sleeping with the back of the body up (and the face facing sideways or downwards).
iii) reading for long hours with face *bent down or*
iv) doing work with a bent neck for a long time.

An inability to lift the hands or pain in the hands may also be due to keeping the neck *bent forward* for a long time. It may also be due to the stooping down of the shoulders or keeping the hands forward for a long time as in the case of typing. Keep the neck straight with reference to the backbone and keep the shoulders raised to avoid straining the nerves passing through neck.

A burning sensation in the food pipe inside the chest two hours after eating may indicate the beginning of diabetes. One should avoid overeating and increase physical activity. A dry mouth or a frequent feeling of thirst after an hour of eating sweets or food may indicate the onset of diabetes.

Children infested with worms sleep with eyes partially open or gnaw their teeth while sleeping. Deworm periodically.

Try to identify the reason and take necessary corrective steps instead of increasing the dosage of medicines.

Inform the doctor by observing the symptoms correctly—just like a sensation in the joints, the increase or decrease of some symptoms while eating some food or doing some activity, etc.—so that the doctor can diagnose the disease correctly.

THE COMMON COLD

Our nose filters the dust, bacteria, virus, etc. in the air, and even after that, some of them enter the lungs. Our lungs try to remove the dust through sneezing or coughing. Even then, some dust, pollen, etc. settle in the moist layers of mucus in the inner walls of the lungs. The common cold is a periodic cleaning of the lungs by our body.

There are more than 200 viruses causing the common cold. The symptoms include nasal discharge, sore throat, cough, and fever. There will be watery nasal discharge initially for a few days followed by a thick discharge of phlegm. It may take about seven days to cure automatically. Since there is no medicine to kill the virus, doctors do not give any medicine for the common cold except for associated side-infections.

Once affected by the common cold, it is better to remove the nasal discharge frequently with the help of a dry kerchief. (Put some oil—like olive oil, coconut oil, etc.—lightly on the nose to minimize skin irritation.) An infected throat may cause serious breathing problems. Gargling* with warm salt-water may help to soothe the sore throat. Clean the mouth with pure water after gargling.

If there is too much congestion of mucus in the air pipe (trachea) or lungs, it will be communicated by our body through fever. Prefer to take common medicines to control fever after consulting a doctor. Taking too many such tablets may damage the kidneys or cause stomach ulcer. Our lungs try to remove the virus, dust, etc. in the lungs through coughing out the dust or virus attached to the mucus.

Sometimes, the intake of too much antibiotics or medicinal foods like ginger causes the porous mucus layer inside the lungs to go dry, and hence make it difficult for oxygen to reach the inner walls of the lungs for absorption in the blood. This causes difficulty in breathing, and sometimes shows asthmatic symptoms. In that case, taking cough syrup or a spoon of honey with warm water may help to make the mucus watery, and remove it through coughing.

Avoid medicines to suppress the symptoms of the common cold which may cause severe side effects, both short-term and long-term. Eat well and take some rest. That will cure the common cold.

If the nasal discharge is greenish or coloured or smells foul, it indicates some kind of infection.

If pollen, dust, or heavy particles lie in the lungs for a long time without being removed by sneezing or coughing, infection of the lungs may occur, and sometimes, it may cause cancer.

DIABETES

Diabetes is neither caused by any virus nor by any bacteria, but by our own lifestyles and eating habits. It is better to guard against it rather than suffer the consequences.

Sugar is an essential food perpetually needed for our body. It is needed for maintaining our body temperature and for doing any work internally, or externally, by our body. Our brain needs continuous supply of sugar (in the form of glucose) and oxygen (a part of air that we breathe) for proper working and maintenance. If it does not get sufficient sugar, as in the case of standing idly for a long time, our brain will order the body to faint so that the head will come down horizontally along with the body. That will help more blood to flow into the brain, and our brain will get enough glucose and oxygen for survival. Lack of glucose and oxygen even for a short time will affect the brain irrevocably.

Sugar and starch are processed in the stomach and intestines and converted into glucose. Glucose is absorbed in the blood and used by the body directly. Insulin produced by our pancreas converts the excess glucose into another chemical called glycogen. Glycogen is stored in the liver, and whenever needed, it is reconverted into glucose by glucagon, another chemical secreted by pancreas, and taken into the blood, and converted to energy using the air inhaled through our nose.

Simply saying, sugar is stored in the liver and is used by our body whenever needed, particularly when we do physical work. If sugar cannot be stored in the liver due to the short production of insulin, then our body will be in a precarious situation and the right amount of sugar has to be eaten regularly and in time.

Blood sugar level in our body will, normally, be around 120 milligrams per decilitre. While getting up from bed in the morning, it will be less. After taking food, it may be more if the excess sugar is not converted into glycogen and stored in the liver. Very less blood sugar will cause dizziness and fainting, if sugar is not stored in the liver. More sugar in the blood will be excreted by the kidneys, if it is not utilised by our body for doing work.

When we eat more sugar and starch at a time or drink more alcohol, the organs processing sugar become overloaded, and just like any overloaded machine, they collapse. Necessary insulin cannot be produced. Unprocessed sugar in the blood cannot be stored in the liver. Physical work may reduce the sugar level in the blood at this stage - after an hour of taking food. Since liver cannot store the excess sugar due to short production of insulin and kidneys will remove it, our body cannot get sugar whenever needed.

More water is needed to excrete more sugar by the kidneys, and so, one may feel more thirsty. Due to overwork, kidneys may fail, particularly if we do not take more water.

After the kidneys fail, wastes like urea in the blood accumulates, and blood pressure develops.

Since sugar cannot be stored or used properly, our body tries to use fat unsuccessfully for energy, and due to the production of more wastes by burning fat and high blood pressure, blood vessels in the heart get affected, causing heart problems.

Diabetes causes the tiny blood vessels in the back of the eye (retina) get blocked, and loss of vision occurs. Nerves also get affected.

Also, there are the non-curable nature of wounds and associated complications due to diabetes.

Why are there so many complications? Our body is meant for active work throughout the day and not for idle life. Use the excess sugar to do more work, particularly physical work.

Eat right amount of balanced food at any time and avoid overloading the stomach with sugar and carbohydrates even though they are essential for maintaining our body and mind or for doing any work. Normally, one takes stomachful of food three times in a day- breakfast, lunch, and dinner. If one does not feel hungry, one should eat after a few hours or skip the next meal. It can be eaten in small amounts many times by patients of diabetes, spread over some intervals, after what was eaten is digested. It takes about three hours to digest a stomachful of normal food. At least once in a day, eat after feeling a little hungry so that different chemicals are secreted by our body to store, and reconvert to, glucose, a form of sugar.

We cannot take insulin with our food. Insulin will get damaged in the stomach due to the acid in the stomach, and it will not reach the blood if taken orally. But our body is a big chemical factory which produces many chemicals including insulin. Which food or which chemical is needed for the production of insulin by our body? Of course, we do not know. So prefer to eat a variety of food in your diet, particularly different types of vegetables and seasonal fruits for a diabetes-free life. Do not be selective in eating food.

Most of the messages inside the body are communicated through many chemicals, including the release of sugar from the liver into the blood. If we take many chemicals, as in the case of medicines and preservatives in packed food, insulin production is likely to be affected. So avoid prolonged use of medicines, which may react with some food producing unwanted chemicals in our body, unless advised by the doctor. Also, use fresh food compared to tinned or packaged food. At least once in a day, eat after feeling a little hungry so that different chemicals are secreted to store the sugar in the liver and to release the sugar in the blood.

Compared to starchy foods (like wheat, rice, corn, millets, roots like potato, etc.), sugar (sweets) will be digested quickly. Compared to sugar(sweets), alcohol(liquor) will be digested quickly in the stomach and absorbed directly into the blood stream. Starchy food will be processed in the body slowly and will get absorbed slowly to suit our body's needs. So prefer starchy food to sugary food. Avoid alcohol unless you are very extremely tired and need instant energy.

Alcohol is directly absorbed from the stomach into the bloodstream, and hence, a lot of sugar will suddenly go into the blood. If the sugar in the blood is not processed in time or used by our body through physical work, the risk of diabetes is more. So avoid liquor or take liquor to the absolute minimum when you are direly in need of instant energy. Take more water with alcohol since more water is needed for digesting it. Since water is also absorbed directly from the stomach whenever needed, it will reduce the strain on the kidneys if it has to excrete the excess sugar. Also avoid taking alcohol(liquor like rum, wine etc.) in empty stomach and prefer to take it with food to avoid problems for liver.

When eating sweets and food with more sugar, eat with different kinds of food to avoid more absorption of sugar at a time.

Sugar in the food gets absorbed in the blood after an hour of taking food. Try to use the sugar in the body by doing some physical and mental work including walking, cycling, etc. *after an hour of taking food* instead of storing it forever for future use.

Instead of using warm water, taking bath in slightly cool water in the morning helps our body to use some extra sugar for the maintenance of our body.

Our lungs and heart are entwined uniquely in supplying oxygen, sugar and other essential nutrients to our body and removing the wastes like carbon dioxide and other chemicals like urea from our body. Non-removal of wastes will shock most of the internal organs including pancreas and liver which process sugar. Sitting idly for a long time will affect the lungs, and hence the heart, resulting in irregular flow of blood to all tissues in our body. That causes non-removal of wastes from all parts of our body besides supplying less oxygen and nutrients to all internal organs which causes improper functioning or malfunctioning of pancreas and liver also. So those whose work involves continuous sittings may prefer to stand up and move a little for about five minutes after every hour so that the blood flow is smooth to all parts. After an hour of taking food, half an hour of physical work will reduce the risk of diabetes very much.

Nasal blockage for a long time, due to allergy, high blood pressure, infection of lungs or throat, polluted environment or due to any other reason, may affect the body metabolism, and hence, less sugar will be used by the body. Such people are more likely to be affected by diabetes unless they are physically active. Nasal blockage due to infected throat is far more serious and its effect can be mitigated by gargling* with warm salt-water.

While standing, take deep breath *towards the forehead* so that the chest and stomach expands, keep it in the lungs for about five seconds, or as long as you can hold breath in the lungs so that the blood flows smoothly throughout the body and then exhale *slowly*. Fast exhalation may cause headache. Do this deep breathing *e*xercise** for about 15 minutes in the morning and evening daily so that the excess sugar is burnt properly. Leave a gap of about 10 seconds between each deep breathing exercise. Those with more blood sugar may do this deep breathing exercise after an hour of taking food also every day. Within 3 days, check the blood sugar level. In case of dizziness or fainting, reduce the medication or the quantity of insulin, and then consult a doctor. Check the blood sugar level every month and reduce or discontinue medication depending on the blood sugar kevel. It may take about 3 to 6 months for the blood sugar level to come to normal level. After reducing the blood sugar to normal level, check the blood sugar every 3 months to monitor whether old life styles have come back.

A burning sensation inside the chest (in fact, it is in the oesophagus, the food pipe from the throat to stomach) after two hours of taking food may indicate the onset of diabetes. Occasional burning sensation may be due to overeating, and people normally use antacids to suppress the symptom.

Dry mouth or a frequent thirsty feeling after an hour of taking sweets or food may indicate the onset of diabetes. Males may experience sexual erection problem.

Those who wake up in the night more than once in the night for urinating may better go for a blood-sugar test. (Sometimes, it may be due to infection in the kidneys also)

What to eat to avoid diabetes? Eat normal food, do deep breathing exercise, and avoid sitting for more than an hour. Eat normal balanced food and avoid enriched food daily. Be physically active throughout the day. Doing hours of morning exercise and living the rest of the day idly will not help to avoid diabetes. As long as physical exercise is not in the form of routine physical work like walking to the market or office, playing with friends, taking your children out for a stroll, etc., the charm for exercise will slowly die.

For those whose lifestyle changes suddenly from an active life to an almost idle life, as in the case of pensioners, sportspersons, etc., it is better to reduce the intake, and the type, of food to avoid diabetes or other diseases.

HIGH BLOOD PRESSURE (HYPERTENSION)

When the heart pumps the blood into the arteries so that it reaches all parts of our body, more pressure is exerted on the blood vessels, called systolic pressure. When it finishes pumping the blood and relaxes to fill itself with blood, the pressure in the arteries will be low, which is called diastolic pressure. Normally, the pressure will be 120/80 which means the systolic pressure is 120 millimetres of mercury and the diastolic pressure is 80. Blood pressure varies from time to time daily, and the tolerable upper limit is 140/90, particularly for old people.

If the pressure is more, the blood vessels sometimes expand to reduce the pressure. In the case of old people, the blood vessels may not expand, causing more blood pressure. Sometimes, plaque due to fatty deposits on the inner side of the blood vessels may cause narrowing of the blood vessels. This also raises blood pressure. Avoid too much of fatty or oily food. Sometimes, nerves also force the blood vessels to contract due to physical or psychological reasons.

When you are taking medicines for high blood pressure, minimise taking fatty foods like mutton to avoid medicinal side-effects which may affect heart.

However, the following causes may cause high blood pressure:

i) mental tension and worries;
ii) strain to the nerves of external organs like the neck, hands, wrists, backbone, etc; or
iii) stress and strain of internal organs like the heart, kidneys, etc.

So, our nerves are directly or indirectly involved in high blood pressure.

Mental tension prepares our body to face an emergency-like situation, and a lot of blood flows in our body to face the situation, imaginary or real. To control high blood pressure, it is better to act according to the perception of mind. Do physical work like running, fast cycling, etc. so that the body can cope with the perceived situation of the mind. Also, try to divert the attention from the cause of worry by singing loudly, talking to good friends, moving on a journey, etc.

Sleep soothes the mind. After doing some physical work and after taking stomachful of food (including an adequate quantity of water), one will surely have sound sleep. Without physical work, one may find it difficult to sleep. Lack of sleep may increase mental tension.

Normally, reading by _bending the neck too much for a long time_ makes the nerves passing through the neck bones (in fact, the meninges or protective membranes covering the nerves) to be pressed while the neck is back to the normal position. This causes high blood pressure. Such people can lay down on the floor or a flat bed with the face up and move the head _slowly_ towards both shoulders without lifting the head for about twenty times. After about ten days, when the strain on the neck eases, keep some weight on the head and move in the room. This may help.

Drooping the shoulders down or moving the hands forward for a long time, as in the case of typing, may cause strain to the nerves passing through the neck and going to the hands. Keep the shoulders raised. Not sitting properly for a long time may strain the nerves going through the backbone. These may cause high blood pressure. So sit properly or do the work in the natural posture or right posture.

Nerves play a major role in monitoring and regulating blood flow. Sitting idly for a long time causes normal blood flow in some portions of the body and reduced blood flow in some portions below the buttocks. This causes strain to the heart and nerves which try to give normal supply of blood to all tissues in the body by pumping more blood forcefully. If the body tissues do not get blood, they will die and nerves, which monitor the blood flow, may behave abnormally. This causes high blood pressure. People whose work involves continuous sitting should stand or move for about five minutes every hour. If the blood pressure is abnormally high, they can do deep breathing exercise** every hour. A strained body for a long time—as in the case of a crouched position or sitting bending the body forward, pressing the stomach—may cause high blood pressure.

Overeating causes more intake of the common salt, and while processing and using more food, more wastes like urea are produced which, in turn, raises the blood pressure. Prefer to do some physical work like running, fast walking, playing, etc. which causes perspiration and hence helps the skin to supplement the kidneys in removing the wastes and the excess common salt. Reduce the amount of food, particularly rich food and enriched food like cheese, sugar, oily food, fried chicken, alcohol, milk powder, sweets, etc., and increase the intake of water.

Also, overeating or having a pot belly causes the expansion and contraction of the diaphragm, a muscular partition separating the chest and stomach, difficult and causes problem in the working of lungs and hence causes improper breathing. This affects the blood pressure.

Stressed internal organs like kidneys, liver, etc. due to overeating specific nutrients may cause high blood pressure. The distress signals may be passed through chemicals which our nerves pick up and respond causing high blood pressure.

Blood pumping is directly related to the lungs and hence to breathing. While standing, take deep breath towards the forehead so that the chest and stomach expand, keep it for about five seconds in the lungs, or as long as you can hold breath so that the blood flows to all parts of the body speedily and then exhale very slowly. Fast exhalation may cause headache. This deep breathing exercise[**] will help in normalising blood pressure, if done for about 15 minutes daily in the morning and evening. Check the blood pressure within two days and reduce the medicines accordingly after consulting your doctor. Those, who continue to take medicines for high blood pressure after doing the deep breathing exercise, may experience low blood pressure, and males may experience sexual erection problem. Check the blood pressure every week and reduce the medicines accordingly. It may take about 3 to 6 months to normalise the blood pressure. After reducing the high blood pressure to normal level, check the blood pressure every 3 months to monitor whether old life styles have come back.

While doing deep breathing exercise, too much expansion of chest may not reduce the blood pressure to normal level and too much expansion of stomach may cause low blood pressure.

Initially, one can stand with the back of the body, heels, and head touching a wall for doing the deep breathing exercise. Once this body posture is known, one can do it anywhere.

The deep breathing exercise helps the expansion, and constriction, of the diaphragm which, in turn, helps digestion and the smooth bowel movement. So, one can avoid constipation and gas trouble. Of course, one may feel more hungry.

Frequent or violent inhalation of air with more chest expansion may increase the systolic pressure while fast exhalation may cause the diastolic pressure to go below normal level. Fast exhalation may also cause headache. Stiff stomach, which normally occurs while in tension, may cause high blood pressure. So, regulate blood pressure through fast work like running, fast cycling, playing, doing heavy work, fast exercise etc.

High blood pressure due to mental tension causes sleeplessness. But high blood pressure due to strained body parts like neck bending, improper posture in sitting, etc. may cause sleepiness. Also high blood pressure causes acute constipation and gas trouble and hence causes sudden eruption of pimples, corn, etc. High blood pressure, in the long run, may damage most of the internal organs of our body. It may cause kidney failure and heart failure or affect the blood vessels in the eyes, brain, etc.

A red tint in the eyes after taking a bath may be due to high blood pressure. A blocked nose may be one of the reasons for high blood pressure. Severe constipation or gas trouble may indicate high blood pressure. Sometimes, in extreme cases, dots of light may appear in the eyes, slowly move, and disappear from the eye while one is awake. Try to avoid high blood pressure, and if diagnosed with high blood pressure, try to identify the causes and avoid life-long medication.

In short, do deep breathing exercise and avoid sitting for more than an hour to avoid high blood pressure.

CANCER

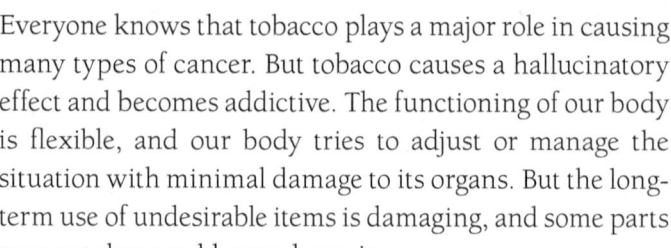

Everyone knows that tobacco plays a major role in causing many types of cancer. But tobacco causes a hallucinatory effect and becomes addictive. The functioning of our body is flexible, and our body tries to adjust or manage the situation with minimal damage to its organs. But the long-term use of undesirable items is damaging, and some parts may get damaged beyond repair.

There are a lot of chemicals in tobacco which cause different types of cancer. So avoid smoking and avoid being nearby smokers while they smoke. Smoking causes lung cancer, cancers in different parts of our body, and other associated diseases. Even though smoking may give pleasure or a sense of company to a smoker, it is better to leave smoking.

Eating or the oral use of tobacco may cause mouth cancer, stomach cancer, or cancer of the food pipe(oesophagus).

Different parts of our body or its components like blood, skin, etc. are replaced or repaired periodically by producing new cells in the required quantity. New cells are produced by dividing a cell into two cells. When new cells are produced in an uncontrolled manner, in general, cancer is caused. Different parts of the body and the cells communicate with each other mostly through chemicals. When the chemical message is blocked or the cell is damaged or manipulated due to the chemicals in the contaminated food and polluted air or water, cancer cells may grow abnormally.

Pesticides in the vegetables or vegetables grown with polluted water may cause cancer since the chemicals in the pesticides may interfere with the functioning of some cells. Pollution in the air or insecticide spray may cause lung cancer.

Our body produces vitamin D through Sunlight. If one is idle under the sun for a long time, sunburn may happen, and in the long run, it may cause skin cancer. So be physically active under the sun so that the water in the perspiration will absorb the sun's ultraviolet rays and heat, and keep the skin cool and healthy.

Even eating only refined food and enriched food (like fried chicken, milk-sweets, cheese, etc.) will cause constipation and, in the long run, will cause colon cancer. That is, even food in excess (more nutrients than necessary) causes cancer. Prefer food prepared in the home to commercially available food.

Eat stomachful of normal food in time to avoid ulcer in the stomach and ulcer, in the long run, causes cancer. The major need of our body is energy to do work and for body maintenance. So the major part of our food should be starchy food which is available in roots, corn, millets, rice, and wheat products with other components like mutton, fat, sugar, vegetables, fruits, etc. in limited quantity.

A long-term use of X-rays or exposure to nuclear radiation may cause blood cancer.

HEART PROBLEMS

All tissues of our body should be supplied with blood continuously, failing which they would die very soon. That work is done by our heart which also supplies blood to itself and it is monitored by the nerves.

When one sits continuously for a long time, pure blood could not be supplied freely below the buttocks, and impure blood cannot reach the heart smoothly. That causes the heart and nerves to strain themselves to supply blood to all parts of the body which causes high blood pressure and other related problems. So avoid a sedentary life and prefer physical work and exercise throughout the day for a good heart. That is, do physical work throughout the day uniformly instead of doing work for an hour and resting throughout the rest of the day.

Our heart does not supply blood uniformly to all parts at all times. When one runs, more blood is supplied to the legs; after taking food, more blood is supplied to stomach; when facing a danger, it pumps more blood to all relevant parts; etc.

Our body needs cholesterol in small quantities which is richly available in animal fats, butter, egg yolk, etc. (If it does not get sufficient cholesterol, it prepares cholesterol for itself from the food we take.) When our body gets more cholesterol but it is not utilised in the form of physical work or when it cannot process fat properly, fine granules of fat get deposited inside the blood vessels, which obstruct the free flow of blood since the blood vessels become narrow. This causes strain to the heart muscles which pump more forcefully. When these fatty deposits become plaque(sticky hardened substance) narrowing the coronary arteries of the heart permanently, the heart muscles strain themselves to pump enough blood, particularly when one does physical work or exercise. This causes coronary heart disease, in which case one gets perspiration and pain emanating from the heart. Those who are physically inactive may prefer vegetable oils to animal fat.

Sometimes, a part of coronary arteries get blocked almost completely due to a blood clot, fat granules, etc. at the site of plaque, resulting in the death of a part of the heart muscles. This causes heart attack (myocardial infarction).

Good sleep is essential so that the heart muscles can take some rest by reducing the workload.

Taking a *clove* of fresh garlic with meals frequently may reduce the risk of the formation of plaque. Fresh vegetables and fruits, which are rich in vitamin C, may also help in reducing plaque formation. But once fat becomes plaque, it is very difficult to remove.

Heart muscles shrink and relax due to electricity produced on the surface of the heart which does not function directly under the nervous system. Of course, nerves can affect the heart indirectly by affecting the electricity-producing tissues. The heart muscles contract the upper and lower chambers of the heart (auricles and ventricles) which causes the heart valves to close at two different times. That makes two different sounds called heartbeat. A rhythmic heartbeat, in all circumstances, means the heart is normal—that is, while physically active, the heartbeat may be more, but the heartbeat cycle is maintained without pain or irregular beating. However, nerves and certain chemicals in the blood can greatly influence the heartbeat and blood supply. Avoid mental tension. Fear and danger may also increase heartbeat by supplying more blood to face the new situation.

Heart function is closely related to the lungs. Improper functioning of the lungs may affect the working of the heart. So avoid smoking, infection of the lungs, infection of the throat, etc.

Bacteria which cause inflammation and pain in the joints may affect the heart valves. Bacteria which cause sore throat may cause inflammation of joints. So keep your mouth clean, and hence the throat, for a good heart.

High blood pressure and diabetes may affect the heart very much.

The heart is one of the important organs in the body and is not the only one. So too much food restrictions or too much medicines for the sake of the heart may affect the health of the other body parts badly.

Heart does its work smoothly when the blood flows smoothly and so, avoid sitting for long hours for a good heart.

BODY: EYE

- Keep your eyes away from heat, particularly hot air. Also, never allow hot water to enter your eyes, particularly while taking a bath in hot water. That may damage the eyes.

- Our eyes are sensitive to light. Never look at intense light like welding sparks, sunlight, etc. directly. That may cause cataract in the eyes and damage the retina in the eye.

- Avoid a sudden change from darkness to light. The pupil in the eye will take some time to adjust to the sudden change. Prefer to close your eyes if you are in a safe place or position.

- Watch television from at least three metres (approximately 10 feet) away from it. Also, keep the room lighted while watching television. That will help to avoid eye strain.

- Taking bath with cool water will help in keeping your eyes and head cool, particularly when you have to do work under the sun. However, dry the hair immediately after taking a bath since prolonged exposure of the head to water may lead to sinusitis which, in turn, may cause headache.

- Food rich in vitamin A, like carrot, sweet potato, milk, butter, egg-yolk, etc., will help your eyes to be healthy.

❖ Good sleep soothes the eyes and helps to ease eye strain. Prefer 8 to 10 hours of sleep daily. Children need 10 to 12 hours of sleep.

❖ Never read anything while lying down on the bed. While reading, keep the book *at least* one foot away. If the light is more or the size of the letters is big, then the distance from the eye should be still more to avoid eye strain and eye defects. Sometimes, one may feel headache, if the book is read by keeping it closely. Mobiles and laptops should be kept approximately two feet away since the letters are bright. Children who play games in the mobiles may keep it close to them and may develop eye defects like short-sight (myopia) later because of which they cannot see objects kept a little away. They may need to wear spectacles in future.

❖ Hold the book in a slope, preferably midway between horizontal and vertical (45 degrees) while reading. If the book is heavy, prefer to bend your body slightly forward to avoid any strain to your neck which may lead to symptoms like spondylitis.

❖ In case any foreign objects like dust enters the eyes, bending downwards, prefer to wink the eyes in a handful of water or wink repeatedly to remove it to a corner and then manually remove it. Rubbing the eyes while dust or sand is inside the eyelids may damage the eyes.

❖ Headache may also be experienced if one uses other's spectacles.

BODY: EAR

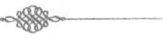

- ❖ Avoid inserting sticks, cotton buds, etc. to clean the ear. They may damage the ear.
- ❖ Ear is sensitive to sound. Keep away from too much sound or noise, particularly drumbeats, loudspeakers, explosions, etc. It may damage the eardrums or create headache or mental perturbation.
- ❖ While suffering from the common cold, if your ear pains, it may be due to an imbalance of air pressure inside the ear. Inhale more air and close your nose with both fingers and close your mouth. Try to exhale air by putting pressure on your nose. It may ease the pain by normalizing air pressure in the ear. Throat infections or nasal blockade may cause an imbalance of air pressure inside the ear. Gargling* with warm salt-water for about five minutes may reduce throat infection and help ease ear pain.
- ❖ While swimming or taking a bath, if water enters the ear and gives pain while moving your head this way or that way later, pour more water into that ear and then empty it by tilting your ear downwards. The water trapped inside the ear will come out and ease the pain.

❖ Ensure that no foreign object enters the ear. In case ants enter the ear, showing light from outside or closing the ear with a hand and removing the hand alternatively may help the ant or insect to find its way out. Otherwise, if the ant does not come out, pour water and then dry it by tilting your head. Avoid inserting sticks or cotton buds to remove it.

❖ Avoid hot water or hot air entering the ears. It may damage hearing.

BODY: NOSE

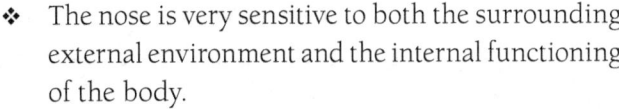

- ❖ The nose is very sensitive to both the surrounding external environment and the internal functioning of the body.
- ❖ If we exclude the balanced food, then most of the health-related problems may be associated with the nose which, in turn, may be related to the throat, lungs, stomach, or to lack of physical work.
- ❖ Avoid places with dirt or impure air or smoke. Otherwise, the lungs may be affected, which may initiate a chain of other symptoms.
- ❖ Nose filters dust, bacteria etc. Always try to inhale air through the nose unless you are short of breath, as in the case of swimming underwater. Inhaling through the mouth may lead to dry cough since dust may enter the lungs and the lungs will try to send them out by violent sneezing. Inhaling through the mouth may also cause throat infection and perpetual cough.
- ❖ A runny nose is a symptom of the common cold. Eat well and take rest and try to dry it out with a kerchief rather than attempting to suppress the symptoms with medicines. It may lead to side effects later.

❖ While suffering from the common cold, the throat is normally infected. Try to gargle[3] with warm salty water. After gargling, clean your mouth with pure water so that more salt does not find its way to your stomach. Some other bacteria in the throat and respiratory tract, which cannot be killed by gargling, can be killed by breathing steam from hot water through the mouth. But never take hot food or hot drinks to soothe the throat. It may damage the teeth or the food pipe(oesophagus). Also, avoid hot dry air.

❖ Never trim the hair inside the nostrils too much. It may lead to more dust particles entering the lungs and the lungs will try to send them out through violent coughing or sneezing.

❖ Frequent sneezing may indicate an allergy. Try to observe whether anything from the air, water, or food is causing the allergy and try to minimize the contact or its use.

❖ Never insert your finger or any foreign object to clean the nose. It may lead to nasal bleeding.

❖ In case you feel sleepy on any occasion when you should be alert or awake, inhale more air, keep it for a few seconds, and then exhale it slowly, simulating active physical work. Avoid this practice for more than five minutes. Better go for a nap, in case one should be alert for more time.

❖ Sitting for long hours or physical inactivity may lead to nasal problem or breathing problem. After

---

[3] Dissolve maximum possible amount of salt in a mouthful of warm water(NOT hot water) and pour it into your mouth. By keeping your face upward, tell 'ha . . . ha . . ha...' for about a few minutes.

an hour of sitting, try to walk or stand up for about five minutes.

- ❖ Drinking water, instead of food, while feeling hungry may cause nasal blockage.

- ❖ Keep away from unpleasant odours. They may not be good for your lungs or for your health.

- ❖ Nasal blockage or lung infection may seriously hinder the physical performance, particularly in games and sports, since one would not get enough oxygen from air to convert the sugar or fat in our body into energy. It may affect joints, particularly neck and backbone if heavy work is done without warming up the body.

- ❖ Too much nasal blockage, throat infection or lung infection will seriously affect the body metabolism, and hence, those with nasal blockage are likely to be affected by diabetes and blood pressure unless they are physically active.

- ❖ When there is nasal blockage, if one stands for a long time idly, the heart may not be able to pump enough blood to the brain. The autocorrect mechanism of the brain may order the body to fall down unconsciously so that enough blood is supplied to the brain. The person who falls down will become normal within a few minutes.

- ❖ Overeating and having a pot belly will affect the expansion of the lungs, and hence, breathing problems may occur.

- ❖ Hot air exhaled, after doing hard work like playing, running, cycling etc, kills some bacteria in the throat and respiratory tract, and also helps to avoid sinusitis. The exhaled hot air helps to evaporate the water in the sinuses, the cavities behind the nose that open into nasal cavities and helps to avoid sinusitis.

❖ Do deep breathing exercise** in the morning and evening to remove the waste stagnant air (carbon dioxide) from the lower part of the lungs.

❖ Sitting idly for long hours daily for months together affects breathing, and it may affect the blood flow to reproductive organs, and it may cause infertility and other problems related to reproductive organs.

❖ If one takes too much antibiotics or medicinal food like ginger, it will dry the mucus lining in the lungs and one may feel breathing problems or experience asthmatic symptoms. In that case, take a spoonful of honey in a glass of warm water. It will make the mucus watery and help to breath normally. Some cough syrups also help.

❖ Nasal blockage or breathing difficulties may lead to the following related problems:
  i) indigestion
  ii) constipation
  iii) gas problems (flatulence) and acute gas problems with rash, pimples, corn, skin diseases, etc.

BODY: MOUTH

❖ The mouth should be wet always. Drink enough water.

❖ After taking food, clean the mouth with water so that bacteria do not thrive on the food particles. In case of sticky food, keeping water in the mouth, use your finger like a brush to remove it, particularly, the food at the end of the wisdom teeth-the last teeth in the mouth. The wisdom-teeth are the neglected teeth in the mouth.

❖ Keeping salty water in the mouth for a few minutes kills many bacteria in the mouth, gums, and teeth. After spitting out the salt-water, ensure that the mouth is cleaned with pure water to avoid any future complication like high blood pressure.

❖ Infection of the gums or teeth will cause infection in the throat. Also, breathing through the mouth will infect the throat. Food particles in-between the teeth help some bacteria to proliferate and they infect the throat also. Gargling* with warm salt-water will kill some of the bacteria in the throat. Gargle when you are having infections like the common cold, cough, tooth-pain, etc. Frequent yawning may indicate that the throat is infected. An infected throat would cause nasal blockage and create gastric problems and other serious undiagnosable symptoms. Severe infection of throat may cause regurgitation, and male persons may experience sexual erection problem. Gargle with warm salt-water to breathe normally.

❖ Hot air exhaled, due to physical work like running, playing etc., kills some other bacteria in the throat and respiratory tract, for which gargling does not work. One has to inhale steam from boiled water through the mouth to kill such bacteria. But never eat hot food or drink hot drinks to soothe the throat. It may damage the teeth or the food pipe(oesophagus). Avoid hot dry air also.

❖ Very hot food may damage the teeth. Very cold food may also damage the teeth. But eating very hot food and very cold food simultaneously may damage the teeth more.

❖ While taking ice cream or hot drinks like coffee, tea, etc., try to take them without coming into contact with the teeth. Also, prefer to take or sip in small quantities so that the tongue can make it warm or cool before gulping it down.

❖ Sticky sweets like chocolates may damage the teeth more if not cleaned very soon. Prefer to take sour items without touching the teeth, if possible, for it may damage the enamel, the outer covering which protects the teeth. So after eating sweets or sour items, prefer to clean the mouth with water.

❖ When food particles are trapped in between the teeth or in between the gums and teeth, some bacteria try to eat and help us. But in the process, they leave some chemicals which cause damage to the enamel or cause tartar (calculus), a hardened sticky substance on the teeth. Thriving under tartar, bacteria damage the teeth further and cause inflammation and bleeding of gums. Sometimes, the gums swell due to infection to get rid of the food particles which causes gum bleeding. So keep the mouth clean, particularly after eating sweets, mutton, etc. Rinse the mouth with water so that food particles attached to the gum and teeth are removed and bacteria may not thrive in the mouth.

❖ Brush the teeth before breakfast in the morning and after dinner in the evening covering *all sides of all the teeth* to remove the tartar and other bacteria. Tartar has to be removed mechanically and not through medicines. Brush the teeth up and down also.

❖ In case food particles are trapped in between the teeth or gums, as far as possible, avoid toothpicks. Prefer to brush it with tooth brush to remove them.

❖ Avoid taking powdered food or spicy hot food or medicines without taking sufficient water. Sticky items and chemicals may create problems in the food pipe (oesophagus).

❖ In case any tooth becomes sensitive while eating sweets or drinking cool water or warm water, consult a dentist.

❖ Avoid licking the lips. That may dry the lips and cause irritation. Applying cooking oil or fat and then cleaning it with cool water may be good for lips.

❖ Vitamin C, which is rich in fresh vegetables and fruits, particularly, citrus fruits, is good for gums. Vitamin C gets almost spoiled if the vegetables or the fruits are boiled or cooked with more heat.

BODY: SKIN

- The major function of the skin in our body is akin to a fort protecting a kingdom and its people from enemies. It stops germs, bacteria, viruses, fungi, etc. from entering our body.

- A damaged skin (due to a fire, injury, etc.) may not be able to filter the germs, bacteria, etc. So protect your skin and maintain it.

- In case a small portion of the skin is damaged due to any scratch or injury, clean it with clean water, dry it with cloth or cotton, and then apply some antibiotic lotion or medicine so that bacteria, viruses, etc. may not enter the body. If nothing is available, apply a little cooking oil or fat.

- Before applying medicine, in case of an injury, ensure that foreign items like dust, sand, broken thorns, etc. are removed from the body. Otherwise, pus will be formed due to infection, and it will take a lot of time for the skin to get itself repaired. Till the foreign object like dust is removed through the pus, the injury will not be cured.

- Heat(hot water, hot oil etc) will damage the skin. In case a major part of the skin is damaged in a fire, keep the skin cool by sprinkling cool and clean water, and then get the services of a doctor.

Never try to remove the sticky items except under the monitoring of a doctor when medicine is applied.

❖ Extreme cold climate may also damage the skin. In that case, enough blood could not be supplied to the skin, particularly to the extremities of our body like the fingers. Physical activity may help blood to flow to all parts.

❖ Sunlight helps the body to prepare vitamin D. So expose your face, bare hands, bare legs, etc. to the sun for about thirty minutes daily. Be active under the sun so that the water in the perspiration absorb the sun's ultraviolet rays and heat, and keep the skin cool. Sitting idly under the sun will damage the skin because of overheating and it may cause cancer in the long run because of sun's ultraviolet rays.

❖ Persistent itching in the skin may be due to the following causes:
   i)   lack of cleanliness in the skin.
   ii) lack of oil in the skin.
   iii) bacterial infection.
   iv) dead skin.

❖ Keep the skin clean including the private parts by taking bath regularly, preferably using soap. Avoid the use of soap in the winter or when the perspiration is less. That will remove the oil on the skin which may cause itching. When perspiration is less, the skin may not get enough oil which it used to get while perspiring even though the sweat and oil glands in the skin are different. Also, new skin is formed every month, and the dead outer layer of the skin is to be removed.

Using soap, while taking a bath, may help to remove the dead skin. Applying oil later will help in stopping itching.

❖ While perspiring, avoid taking bath or washing the face. The pores in the skin might have expanded, and taking a bath immediately will help the skin absorb more water. That will create headache or a feeling of heaviness, or one may be affected with the common cold very shortly. Prefer to wipe off the perspiration with dry cloth or towel.

❖ Cleanliness helps in avoiding contagious diseases. But do not be obsessed with too much cleanliness. Perspiration, dust, bacteria, etc. are normal in life. Even the water that we clean our hands may have bacteria since there is no antibiotic which kills all bacteria. The air that we breath in may have bacteria, pollutants etc.

❖ In case of any inflammation or swelling of the skin, never apply heat nor give hot-water treatment. Clean it with soap and water and then apply some antibiotic powder or lotion, after drying the skin.

❖ In case of boils or swellings, apply medicine without damaging the boils or swellings. That may help to cure faster without much problem.

❖ Skin slowly absorbs liquids from outside. So avoid contact with dirty water or poisonous liquids for long hours.

❖ The skin removes wastes from the body through perspiration. So physical work will help to reduce the strain on the kidneys.

❖ Clean your face with soap daily in the morning and evening so as to avoid pimples. Applying facial creams to avoid perspiration may cause headache. Prefer to wipe the perspiration off the face with a dry kerchief or a towel.

❖ Apply a little oil daily in the lower part of the legs to avoid the formation of scales.

❖ Constipation and gas trouble will cause the formation of pimple-like swellings, corn-type inflammation, skin diseases, etc. So avoid overeating. Avoid high blood pressure.

❖ Vitamin A helps in maintaining the skin which is rich in carrot, spinach, sweet potato, milk, butter, egg yolk etc.

BODY: NECK

❖ Our neck is made of seven bones (cervical vertebrae) with a hole (vertebral foramen) in the centre. Through the hole of the neck bones, the spinal cord, a part of the nervous system, passes. A displaced nerve or strained nerve due to any misalignment of the neck bones may create undiagnosable symptoms including high blood pressure.

❖ The neck should be straight with reference to the backbone—that is, slightly bent forward. Never tilt your neck downwards too much for *a long time*, particularly while reading. Neck pain, stiff neck, or spondylitis may occur. Read books by keeping them at least one foot away and by keeping them in a slope (45 degrees from the vertical).

❖ While reading heavy books, prefer to bend your body forward so that the neck will be straight with reference to the backbone. Also, keep your elbows on the table and hold the book. If the hands are supported on the table, the strain on the nerves through the neck to the hands will be less.

❖ 'Push-up exercise'[4], may help to relieve the strain in the neck immediately by helping to move more blood through the neck.

❖ *Neck exercise:* In case there is pain in the neck or stiff neck or pain in the hands for no reason, prefer to lay down on a flat bed or the floor with the face up and move the head from right to left and vice versa *slowly* for about twenty times without lifting the head. In general, the neck pain is because of the pressure given to the nerves in the neck due to wrong postures. This neck exercise can also be done by standing, with the neck, back, and the heels touching a wall.

❖ In case of stiff neck or neck pain, after doing the above neck exercise for about ten days and *after the pain or stiffness disappears*, prefer to carry a reasonable weight (10 kg to 30 kg) on the head and walk for a few minutes in a room balancing the weight on the head. That may regulate some strained nerves.

❖ While sleeping with the face up, avoid pillows. While sleeping with face sideways, use a pillow of appropriate height and avoid thick pillows.

❖ *Never sleep with your back up* and your face down. This posture may cause stiff neck or spondylitis-like symptoms.

❖ Keep your shoulders raised. Drooping shoulders may strain the nerves passing through the neck, particularly the nerves going to the hands. Also,

---

[4]   Facing the floor, keep both legs and hands on the floor with the body in a flat position. Move the body up and down with hands and keep the body and leg straight.

moving the shoulders forward for a long time, as in the case of typing, may strain the nerves through the neck.

❖ A strained nerve in the neck may cause pain in the hand while lifting a hand or it may immobilise the hands. In that case, do the above neck exercise.

BODY: BACKBONE

The backbone is made up of many small bones with sponge-like cartilage in between them to help for the smooth movement. Through the centre of these bones (vertebral foramen), the spinal cord, a part of the nervous system, passes. If a displaced bone or slipped disc (cartilage) presses the spinal cord, it may have debilitating effect and unbearable pain on the body. So avoid thick mattresses or an uneven bed for sleeping which may displace a disc, pressing the spinal cord and causing serious pain.

Avoid lying down or sitting down on the mattress *violently* since the backbone discs may move from the normal position, severely straining the nervous system passing through the backbone.

Also, avoid jerking or rough-riding while driving any vehicle. Also, avoid starting or stopping any vehicle suddenly while driving. It may also damage the disc or cause disc slippage and cause serious pain on the back or in the neck.

Do some physical work or simple exercise to warm up your body before doing any heavy work. That will help to avoid disc slippage and consequent pain in the backbone.

BODY: INTERNAL ORGANS

All internal organs are closely packed inside our body. In case of rough-riding or jumping from some height, they may hit each other, causing injury. In case of rough-riding for a short while, one can inhale more air and keep it in the lungs for some time so that the organs are more tightly packed, avoiding unnecessary injury or painful rubbing.

Heart: The heart pumps blood throughout the body, including itself. Avoid too much of food rich in animal fat which may block the blood flow in the body by thin granules of fat. Those with less physical activities may prefer vegetable oils to prepare food compared to animal fat.

Sitting idly for long hours may result in free blood flow to most parts and less blood supply to other parts of our body below the buttocks due to pressed blood vessels. This will lead to strained heart and nerves which may cause more heart problems. Every hour, stand up and walk for about five minutes.

An infected throat may affect the joints which, in turn, may affect the heart. So keep your mouth neat and clean to avoid the infection of the throat. Also, avoid inhaling through the mouth.

Smoking will cause narrowing of the blood vessels which may create heart problems.

While doing hard work or while inhaling more air and keeping it in the lungs for a few seconds, if the heart beats irregularly (palpitation) or if a sense of pain is felt, there is some problem in the heart.

Shortage of Vitamin B affects nerves, and hence it may affect the heart. So take sufficient whole grain, milk, green leafy vegetables, legumes, peas, nuts, milk, egg, animal organs like liver, etc.

Fresh vegetables and fruits which are rich with Vitamin C may indirectly help the heart to function properly by its antioxidant properties. Boiling vegetables and fruits will damage Vitamin C.

Lungs: Our lungs are moist chambers which should be kept moist. If the mucus layer in the lungs becomes dry, it will become like a membrane, not allowing air to pass to the sacs (alveoli) in the lungs which exchange oxygen with carbon dioxide in the blood. So our body cannot absorb enough oxygen, and breathing problems or symptoms of asthma may occur. So while having the common cold, avoid too much antibiotics including medicinal food like ginger which will dry the porous mucus layer. (Ginger and other spices are essential for our body.) In case of minor breathing problems, take a simple cough syrup or a spoon of honey with a glass of water for a few days, which will make the mucus or phlegm watery. That will help to remove mucus from the lungs by frequent coughing and make the breathing easy.

Non-absorption of enough oxygen due to a dry mucus layer may seriously affect the body's metabolism, and hence, a sense of 'not willing to do any work' will be in the mind. Of course, our body cannot do any work without the energy produced by the sugar in the food and oxygen in the air.

The lungs are very sensitive to foreign objects like dust, pollen, etc. The lungs will try to remove them by sneezing or through phlegm by coughing. If foreign objects like dust, talcum powder, pollen, asbestos, etc settles down in the lungs, and if they are not removed by coughing, it may lead to infection and, in the long run, sometimes cause cancer. So, avoid suppressing the symptoms like coughing without knowing the reason.

Chemicals in pollutants, chemicals in pesticides, and smoke from burning objects may seriously affect the lungs. In case of a fire, carbon monoxide, a part of partly burned smoke may be absorbed in the blood through lungs and it may cause sudden death.

Smoking tobacco products like cigarettes seriously affects the lungs, sometimes settling down on sacs (alveoli) in the lungs, causing cancer.

Since the inner part of the lungs is not connected to nerves, no pain will be felt before any infection becomes serious.

The diaphragm, a curved muscular layer separating the chest cavity and the abdominal cavity, is compressed downwards when the lungs expand and then expands upwards, forcing the lungs to shrink. This helps in breathing. When one overeats or when one is having a pot belly, the diaphragm cannot expand and shrink properly, causing breathing problems and associated undiagnosable symptoms. The expansion and constriction of diaphragm also helps a lot in digestion and in the smooth bowel movement. Sitting idly for a long time, and mental tension, also affect the functioning of diaphragm. Deep breathing exercise** helps the diaphragm to compress downwards and move upwards.

Waste air (carbon dioxide) being heavy, it tries to settle down in the bottom of the lungs. Deep breathing exercise helps to remove the waste air from the lungs and to absorb pure air (oxygen).

Kidneys: Kidneys remove wastes from our body through urine.

Excess urination may be due to the following causes:

i)   removal of excess sugar which our body cannot process or use.
ii) removal of excess common salt and other wastes produced while processing or using food by our body.
iii) removal of excess food rich in protein (meat, fish, etc.).
iv) removal of excess or unwanted chemicals in the medicines.
v)   removal of poison from the body which normally occurs when we take spoiled food. In all the above cases, not drinking sufficient water may damage the kidneys. Sometimes, kidney stones may be formed.

Some of the sugar is processed and stored in the liver, and some of the sugar is in the blood temporarily for use by the body. If more sugar is in the blood, the kidneys try to remove it. So, avoid taking more sweets and alcohol.

Our body needs common salt. While our body uses food, wastes like urea are produced in the body. When we take more amount of common salt or when we overeat food which produces more wastes, our kidneys try to remove them.

Even though sugar and fat can be stored in our body, there is no place to store excess protein (pulses, meat, cheese, etc.). The kidneys remove the excess protein and other unstorable nutrients. Avoid overeating rich foods like fish, meat, etc. Also, more wastes are produced while using protein which are also to be removed by the kidneys.

An overdose of medicines causes more chemicals in the blood, which our kidneys try to remove. Since a lot of chemicals are absorbed from a single dose of medicine, it will strain the kidneys too much when one takes an overdose of medicines.

It also removes poison from the body. So avoid spoiled food. Also, avoid acidic food (having sour taste like lime juice) kept for a long time in *metallic vessels*. The acid in the food would react with the metal in the vessels and produce poisonous chemicals. Prefer to store acidic food in glass, plastic, or china-clay, bottles. Also, avoid keeping liquid sugar in metallic vessels for a long time which may turn sour due to fermentation.

For removing wastes or excess nutrients and chemicals, the kidneys need a lot of water. So drink enough water. Kidney stones may be formed when we take rich foods and when we do not take sufficient water. Also, the kidneys would strain themselves to remove the wastes like chemicals, poison, etc., and overstrained kidneys may collapse.

Also, not drinking enough water may cause kidney infection. In that case, the urine may become yellowish. Drink more water to wash away the bacteria through urine.

In extreme cases, if there is an acute shortage of water in the body, our body will try to provide water by converting the blood into water, called dehydration. The urine will become yellowish orange (amber) colour, in that case. Drink sufficient water to avoid dehydration.

Stomach: The stomach produces acid to digest the food that we eat. So prefer a stomachful of food when hungry rather than a frugal amount of rich food. Eating small amounts of food may cause the release of more acid in the stomach which may aggravate hunger or one may feel hungry very soon.

For digesting food, the stomach needs water, and so leave enough space for water while eating.

Avoid medicines on an empty stomach including medicinal foods like ginger, pepper, etc. since they may damage the mucus-like linings which protect the stomach from its own secretion of acids. It may lead to ulcer.

After taking food, the stomach needs more blood to constrict and expand and digest the food. So avoid very hard work like running a race or doing strenuous physical work after eating stomachful of food. In case one has to do very hard physical work, one can eat only half stomachful of food.

Avoid rough-riding after the stomach is full which may damage the diaphragm or hit other internal organs, causing swellings.

A spasm of the diaphragm may cause hiccups. Avoid external stress on the stomach, like allowing any child to play on the stomach while lying down on the bed, which may irritate the diaphragm.

BODY: GENERAL

❖ Those who type a lot should type not with the tips of the fingers but tap with the inside ends of the fingers. The nerve endings may cause a painful sensation, particularly, in the winter.

❖ After taking a bath, apply oil to the hair on the head *after* it dries. Otherwise it may lead to frequent cough with small amounts of phlegm coming from the throat.

❖ While walking upstairs or downstairs, always walk with the toe landing first (and heels later) so that it gives some spring effect to the body. That puts less stress on the joints. Also, while jumping, land with the toes first.

❖ The best medicine for a headache is sleep. Sometimes the headache may be due to improper breathing. In that case, take deep breath, hold it for about 5 seconds in the lungs, and then release it slowly. After about 5 minutes of doing this exercise, the headache may disappear. Otherwise, press your temples (small depressions between the eyes and ears) with your fingers to get a temporary relief. If the headache persists, consult a doctor.

❖ Irregular breathing, particularly, fast exhalation of air for sometimes may cause headache. While standing, take deep breath, keep it for about 5 seconds and exhale *slowly*.

❖ While suffering from fever or any kind of sickness, try to eat almost normally even though you do not feel like eating anything. Otherwise, you may feel very weak and unable to do normal work after the recovery from the illness.

❖ If one has to stand for long hours, prefer to move your legs up and down so that blood will not stagnate in the bottom of the legs which may cause pain. Also, idly standing for long hours will result in less blood flow to the brain, which may result in fainting and falling down for a few seconds till the blood supply is normalized in the brain.

❖ Avoid sitting for long hours with the bottom of the thighs pressed with a chair or sofa. The veins in the bottom of the legs may not be able to send the impure (deoxygenated) blood to the heart. The impure blood may stagnate in the veins of the legs for a long time, and the veins may expand beyond its elastic limit, causing varicose veins.

❖ Avoid lifting heavy items with one or two fingers, for it may strain the nerves.

❖ A displaced nerve may cause more pain. So while massaging, apply the pressure along the length of the body, keeping the body in a normal position.

❖ Our nerves, joints, and muscles need warmth. So before doing any heavy work, warm up your body by doing simple exercises or by walking, slow running, etc.

SLEEP

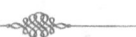

Sleep is an elixir in life which soothes the body and mind. For a sound sleep, sufficient physical activity is essential, and the mind should be free from tension. Without enough sleep, the mind is charged, and it rarely comes to equilibrium which is essential for doing any meaningful activity.

Just like the duration of the day and night varies in a year, the duration of sleep may vary, but within a range, for a normal person. A person without enough sleep is likely to do more mistakes in his activities than a person who has sound sleep. Also, without sleep, one cannot do any mental work, and even if one tries to do, it may not come to fruition or it may take abnormally more time than required. A student is more likely to forget what he has studied within a few days, if studied without sufficient sleep. Less sleep may cause more irritation, particularly, when they hear noise or repeated sound.

The duration of sleep required for human beings varies from age to age—slowly decreasing as the age increases—or as physical activity decreases. However, a normal adult needs approximately eight to ten hours of sleep each day. A school-going child may need around ten to twelve hours of sleep, and an infant may need as much time as it sleeps without being disturbed. An old person who does not do sufficient physical work may not be able to sleep for more than six hours.

Tiredness or fatigue due to physical work helps in getting sound sleep. It is better to do physical work, which needs less concentration of the mind, when one does not have enough sleep. It may not be possible to concentrate on mental work, or the precise handling of physical work when one does not have enough sleep. Children not having sufficient sleep will not be good in their studies, for they cannot be attentive in the class. Sleeplessness may cause more mistakes in doing work and hence more tension.

Sleeplessness may cause headache. Mental tension causes sleeplessness. Acute sleeplessness for a long time may cause serious psychological disorders. Sleeplessness is a major cause for highway accidents.

Negative experiences disturb the sleep very much. So keep away from bad company and avoid doing wrong things.

Avoid taking tea or coffee after dinner. It may cause sleeplessness in the night. Taking more than three cups of tea or coffee during the day may also affect sleep.

A person who cannot sleep while in bed may close the eyes and lay down on the bed without trying to think about anything or meditating on any one thing. On the next day, it is better to do physical work which does not involve minute handling of any work.

HEALTHY LIFE

Health is an important yardstick of living. A healthy mind and a healthy body of a person may enrich one's life besides being productive and useful.

Most of the health-related problems may be attributed to the following causes:

i)   overeating.
ii) eating only selective food.
iii) not removing the waste products from the body *in time*.
iv) lack of physical work.
v)   inhaling stale or polluted air.
vi) not drinking enough water.
vii) lack of sleep.
viii) taking unwanted chemicals, particularly medicines which cause side effects.

Avoid overeating, which would harm health. Avoid an overdose of medicines and try to avoid tinned food which may contain more chemicals as preservatives. The chemicals may affect the functioning of our internal organs which function or react based on chemical cues.

Keep your body neat and clean. Prefer to use soap while taking a bath, particularly if the body perspires in the day. In case of less perspiration, as in the case of winter, avoid soap since it may cause an urge to scratch the skin frequently. In that case, apply a little oil on the skin. The skin is like a fort which keeps the germs off. Many bacteria and viruses enter our body through damaged skin.

Waste is a by-product of any useful work. When we overeat, more chemical wastes, like urea, are produced while processing and using nutrients. The wastes should be removed in time through the nose, kidneys, skin, and anus. Wastes from our body like stool and urine should be removed in time, particularly before taking breakfast. Solid waste and gas in the intestines (flatulence), if mixed with blood, may lead to skin diseases and other undiagnosable symptoms. Also, before taking stomachful of food like lunch or dinner, go to urinal so that the gas in the intestines are released smoothly.

Prefer free-flowing air and avoid closed air for long hours. Ensure that, even in severe winter or hot summer, the windows are kept open for some time and the house is ventilated daily. Avoid inhaling insecticide sprays. Stale air or polluted air should be avoided.

Different types of organs need different types of food for maintenance and functioning. For example, the brain may need sugar, the skin may need oil and water, the blood may need iron, the bones may need calcium, the flesh in the body may need protein, etc. No single food contains everything needed for each organ in the body in required quantities. So prefer to eat a variety of food including seasonal fruits and vegetables. Overeating any food including nutritious food will create a lot of problems for our body.

Physical work or exercise makes the blood flow to different organs in sufficient quantities, gives enough food and energy to all organs, and removes wastes produced in different organs. That keeps all organs healthy and vibrant besides helping them function properly. Without physical work, one may find it difficult to sleep in the night. Prefer to do some productive work in the house or outside including playing rather than doing some exercise.

Go to sleep in time. An adult may need eight to ten hours of sleep. A child may need more sleep, and an old and inactive person may need six to eight hours of sleep. A good sleep refreshes the body and mind. Prefer a physically and mentally active life which would give you sound sleep compared to a sedentary and lazy life.

Avoid tension. Never worry about what you cannot do. If unavoidable, be prepared to bear it or avoid it. But what you can do, delve into it in time with a little planning. Tension can affect our internal organs badly, particularly through excited nerves and blood pressure.

Sunlight is an important aspect of healthy life. Ensure that some parts of the body, like face, bare hands and legs, etc., are exposed to sunlight for at least fifteen minutes, preferably thirty minutes daily. That will help our body prepare the necessary vitamin D and help inhale warm air. Remember that sunlight is also a disinfectant. Lack of exposure to sunlight will lead to symptoms which are difficult to diagnose.

Water is also very essential for maintaining the body and its organs. So prefer to drink enough water after taking food to avoid the formation of stones in the internal organs. Water is also essential for maintaining the body temperature and removing the waste produced in the body through perspiration, urine, and stool. Not drinking sufficient water may cause uncontrolled flatulence and severe constipation. Prefer water compared to carbonated drinks.

Never ask for any immediate cure for your illness from your doctor. An overdose of medicines may induce serious side effects immediately or later in life. Most of the serious illnesses in young age may be attributed to medicinal side effects or overdose of medicines, including medicines to suppress symptoms of the common cold.

Deworm your intestines whenever needed since the worms may eat the essential nutrients needed by the body.

Where mosquitoes are prevalent, prefer to use mosquito-nets while sleeping to avoid diseases like malaria, dengue, encephalitis, yellow fever, etc.

Prefer a physically, and mentally, active life which would give you sound sleep compared to a sedentary and lazy life.

Briefly speaking, a variety of food and good supply of pure air(oxygen) keep our body healthy.

MAINTENANCE OF THE BODY

Maintenance of the body is as important as maintaining a machine, simple or sophisticated.

Our body needs a variety of food including vegetables, greens, and seasonal fruits for growth as well as for the maintenance of our body. General requirements are pure air to breathe and pure water to drink.

Our body needs sleep to give the different tired organs rest or to reduce the work load, particularly that of the brain, heart, eyes, skin, etc.

For the proper functioning of different organs, physical work like walking, playing, exercise, etc. which keeps the body with an abundant blood supply is necessary. Blood supplies the nutrients to all parts of our body and removes the waste produced by them.

Each organ is sensitive to certain factors. The eye is sensitive to light. Avoid seeing intensive light like sunlight, welding sparks, etc. The ear is sensitive to sound. Avoid hearing high decibel noise or loud sound. The skin is sensitive to heat. Avoid burns or avoid standing under sunlight *idly* for a long time. Exposing the body to icy weather may affect the extremities of the body like fingers besides depleting the stored energy from our body. The nose is sensitive to the external environment and internal functioning of our body. Avoid polluted air. The teeth are sensitive to very hot and very cold food. Keep the temperature of food nearer to the temperature of the body while eating. Our body is maintaining itself in a constant temperature. So it is sensitive to extreme heat or cold.

Another important aspect is the *timely* disposal of the waste produced by the body. Ensure that the perspiration in the skin is removed daily by taking bath, preferably using soap in summer. Avoid using soap, if there is less perspiration during the day. Also, the face can be washed with soap twice daily in the morning and evening. Oil can be applied over the skin if the body does not perspire during the day as in winter or if there is an itching feeling in the skin.

Ensure that urine is removed from the body periodically. Ensure that urine is removed before taking food. That will help to relax the muscles and help to release flatulence. Do physical work, like walking, playing, etc., which causes perspiration so that the skin helps the kidneys in removing some waste.

Not releasing flatulence in time may result in the waste gas mixing with blood, and that may cause skin diseases like corn, pimples, etc. and may cause symptoms which are difficult to diagnose. Ensure that you do not sit for long hours, which block the movement of waste gas downwards.

The excretion of solid waste (faeces) from the body daily before taking breakfast is essential for maintaining the body properly. Ensure that you go to the urinals and then drink a glass of water before going to empty the solid waste. That will help to avoid constipation and other related skin diseases and certain undiagnosable symptoms. While standing, take deep breath towards your forehead so that the chest and stomach expands, keep it for about five seconds, and then exhale slowly. Doing this breathing exercise for about 15 minutes daily in the morning and evening may help to avoid constipation. Give a gap of ten seconds between successive deep breathing exercises**. Also taking a small piece of ginger, or food cooked with ginger, at least monthly once, may help to avoid hard motion. Avoid taking too much ginger at a time which may cause breathing problem, if the lung is infected.

Removing the waste air (carbon dioxide) from the blood and taking in pure air (oxygen) is essential for the maintenance of our body. Do physical work or do some exercise which helps to expand and shrink the lungs properly which, in turn, helps to inhale pure air and exhale waste air.

Water helps in moving the food to different parts of the body and removing the waste besides maintaining body temperature. Hence, drink an adequate amount of water, particularly after taking food and in between meals. Not drinking an adequate amount of water may lead to the malfunctioning of the different parts of our body besides causing the formation of stones in different organs in our body.

Mental worries and tension affects all internal organs. So never worry about what you cannot manage.

MARRIAGE

The institution of marriage was started by our forefathers throughout the world since some males did not own the responsibility of fatherhood. Thus, the ceremonies associated with marriage were an implied public declaration by the bride and the bridegroom about a new relationship and the readiness to own all responsibilities of parenthood.

Marriage is the first attempt to live a cooperative living in life by an individual. The bonds connecting life before marriage are loose and flexible, with the necessities of life being made available easily by parents and friends and each one lives a life with less responsibility. With marriage, a new bond is made with responsibility, both implicit and explicit.

As per the law of nature, any man is free to cohabit with any other woman and vice versa. But to bring responsibility and accountability in the conduct of men and women in the society, our elders have introduced the concept of family as a functional unit of society with marriage as the initiation ceremony. Even though the laws of nature often override the implicit and explicit rules and conduct of marriage, the institution of marriage has survived throughout the world.

The institution of marriage fails when men and women become extremely selfish and ignore the responsibility towards the family, particularly towards their spouse and children.

Marriages may be made in heaven, but it hardly stays there. The gravity of nature is so great that the husband and the wife are torn apart physically and psychologically in different directions depending on the physical and psychological needs of the time. Strangely, what one saw as pleasant and alluring before marriage looks differently on close scrutiny. Only the marriages where spouses adjust and cooperate with each other succeed in preserving the family. When the partners go to the extent of illogical limits in disagreeing and conduct themselves accordingly, marriage fails irrevocably.

Strangely enough, man and woman of the same mentality never get married. While the world appreciated the wisdom of Socrates, Xanthippe, his wife, rarely had anything to do with his wisdom.

Man and woman being social animals, the urge to live together as a unit of society is natural. But only when they live together responsibly, the family flourishes in a happy atmosphere.

An ideal family is the one in which the husband and the wife play their roles responsibly for the common welfare of the family, within the limits of permissible deviations. Most of the rules of marriage and family are implicit depending on the society and the mental maturity of the partners in life.

A free discussion about each other's views and activities on each day may help to live a happy life. Do not let the frailties of the human mind spoil marriage, an established institution of society.

In a family, none wins permanently. Sometimes, the other partner may also have a trump card which may turn down one's opinion. Listen to the other side before taking any major decision, whatever your decision would be. But never harp on what cannot be undone.

MARRIAGE: COMPLETION

Both man and woman are incomplete, physically or psychologically. One cannot live without the other. There is always a vacuum in life created by both physical and psychological needs. The institution of marriage tries for the completion of the incomplete man and woman in the society.

Strangely enough, a man or woman of the same nature rarely comes for communion with the opposite sex in any marriage, whether providential marriage, love marriage, or arranged marriage.

Magnetic poles or electric charges of the same kind repel each other, and unlike charges or unlike poles attract each other. As in nature, men and women of the same attributes rarely come together in marriage, whereas men and women of different nature who adjust with, and accommodate to, each other live happily.

A moody person gets a talkative person as a spouse; a wealthy man may prefer a beautiful poor lady for marriage; a beautiful lady may prefer an educated man as her spouse; an artist may prefer an admirer for marriage; a wise person may prefer a pragmatic spouse; a realist may prefer a person who would offer the necessities for his comfortable life; etc.

Far more than anything, it is the behaviour and tone of the speech that determines whether marriage is a completion—that is, whether marriage is made for each other or not. Remember that both behaviour and the way of talking depends on the upbringing by the parents, the status in the society, and the dreams cherished by the person.

With everyone being born selfish, each person wants to gain even in marriage. So you have to give something to your partner in life while getting back something you need from your partner. In marriage, none is a perpetual donor, physically or psychologically. So dreaming of fairies donning out sweeties perpetually and living happily forever is neither feasible nor realistic. A marriage survives in a happy atmosphere only when both partners feel that they have gained, materially or psychologically.

So if you want to live happily, never forget to give something to your spouse—it may be as small as a gem or as big as a sweet word. That fills the vacuum at that moment and makes the life partner feel complete and happy.

SEX AND MARRIAGE

Even though man and woman are physically and psychologically different, they are attracted towards each other naturally by the urge for sex. Compared to material comfort and external behaviour of each other, sexual equation plays a major role in keeping the family atmosphere warm and pleasant. Sexual imbalance may wreck the peace of mind in both partners, and consequently, it may seriously damage the children psychologically. On many occasions, it would cost the happiness associated with marriage forever.

For a good sexual life,

i) spend sufficient time with your spouse and family.
ii) go to bed earlier.
iii) have good and sufficient food daily and in time.
iv) lead a tension-free life.
v) talk freely on all topics, particularly the day-to-day activities, unless it is misused to bully you.
vi) eat a variety of food including all types of vegetables and seasonal fruits.

Nature has set different rules for both man and woman regarding sex. Maintain uniformity and understand the limitations of both males and females.

Since sex is paramount in family life, any denial without proper reason may lead to major misunderstanding and suspicion which, in turn, may lead to abnormal behaviour or serious mental disorder. Try to understand the behaviour of your life partner since, in general, behaviour is a manifestation of the mind in visual form.

Just like hunger, the urge for sex peaks cyclically. So have a faithful partner for life. It is good to be trusted. So be trustworthy.

Sexual performance may be severely affected due to

i)   mental worries and tension.
ii) infection of the lungs, throat or nasal blockage.
iii) low blood pressure or diabetes.
iv) improper functioning of the internal organs.

Doing deep breathing exercises[5] daily for about 15 minutes in the morning and evening and eating a clove of fresh garlic regularly may help in enhancing sexual performance. Avoid doing this exercise while lying down on the bed since more blood may flow to the head, which may cause headache. Also, avoid doing the exercise while sitting since it may affect the heart. Also, while having the common cold or lung infection, taking antibiotics or medicinal foods like ginger which dry the mucus in the lungs may cause poor performance in sex unless taken together with cough syrup or honey.

Sitting idly for long hours daily for years together may affect the blood flow to relevant organs and women may develop menstrual problems and men may develop sexual

---

[5]   While standing, take a deep breath by inhaling more air towards the forehead. Keep it for 5 seconds or as long as you can hold the breath in the lungs and then exhale it *slowly*.

arousal problems. Do deep breathing exercise[**] daily to avoid most problems related to reproductive organs. Also, take a variety of food.

Overindulgence in sex may affect nerves which, in turn, may affect other internal organs in the long run.

MARRIAGE AND ADULTERY

Marriage implies invisible boundaries with implicit rules and trust in following those rules. But nature does not recognize the man-made boundaries. The invisible boundaries of marriage are crossed with impunity by both men and women.

Strangely enough, nature leaves a trail of the breach of trust, but even then, marriage survives by giving the benefit of the doubt or by the law of nature which intertwines men and women physically and psychologically. Since proving adultery is difficult, it starts as suspicion, and as the suspicion appears to be true to a spouse, a storm brews up in the mind and it blows away the near and dear ones, leaving a devastated family.

Men and women who are physically idle or those who are feeling lonely are prone to commit adultery. Since adultery of a spouse has serious impact in the mind, it leads to avenging the betrayal by leading an open life of adultery and immoral behaviour. This has serious impact on all, particularly the children and the society. It affects the self-esteem of the children, and consequently, their life becomes stunted.

Both man and woman are fallible. Before committing adultery, think about the moral responsibility that you owe to your children and the trust that your spouse and children have on you and the untrustworthy moral character of the person with whom you try to have a relationship and the impact that it would have on the family as a whole.

What is traitor to a country, it is adultery to a family. Are you playing your role as a father or mother responsibly? Remember that lions prefer to die for their harems rather than coexist with a rival male. The fate of the cubs may be pathetic.

Having multiple partners may lead to acquiring many sexually transmitted diseases including AIDS. The symptoms of sexually transmitted diseases normally manifest in three days and disappear, but it will reappear and persist after forty days. It is better to consult a doctor after four days. The incubation period for HIV viruses causing AIDS may vary from three months to six months after which one will test positive for AIDS. Lymph nodes may be enlarged within a month of infection by HIV virus. So be faithful to your spouse. Learn to control your sexual urge when needed. An inconspicuous environment for adultery does not guarantee a safe body or mind.

A HAPPY MARRIED LIFE

Immediately after marriage, be polite and considerate and try to understand your spouse. Remember that each one is brought up in a different way. This is particularly true when the spouse comes from a different background—social, economical, or psychological.

Talk freely about your activities, experiences, etc. unless exploited by your spouse. Try to talk from your heart and never be diplomatic. Your spouse can easily find the reality, and that is the beginning of fractures in the relationship. Be frank and avoid hiding relevant facts while speaking.

While your spouse is firm in doing or not doing something, yield to that wish even though it is not correct or appropriate provided that this type of incidents are not frequent. Never forget to counsel later, when your spouse is calm and receptive, if you disagree with your spouse.

Go to sleep earlier. Sleep keeps your body and mind in a refreshed condition. Also, keep your private parts clean by taking bath regularly. Take balanced food (a variety of food including millets, pulses, greens, seasonal fruits, berries, and vegetables) to avoid infertility-related problems.

Never deny sex unless there is any serious problem, physical or psychological. Remember that sex is an important aspect of married life. Prefer a reasonable gap which keeps the body and mind in the right condition. But abstinence or denying sex for a long time may lead to doubts, illusions, or even adultery.

Overindulgence in sex may affect the nerves in the long run. Hence, one can plan according to the body rhythm of one's wife. From the start of the menstrual cycle, the eggs of women may be ready for fertilization for three days, mostly between the thirteenth day and sixteenth day—approximately in the middle of the menstrual cycle depending on the duration of the menstrual cycle. The menstrual cycle starts from the starting day of bleeding. During menstrual period, avoid sex. The body temperature of a woman will also be slightly above normal when the chance for pregnancy is more. Very rich foods and medicines may affect the menstrual cycle which is normally twenty-eight to thirty days. Those who do not plan a child can avoid sex between the tenth day and eighteenth day of the menstrual cycle.[6] Of course, this is not applicable to women having irregular periods.

In the modern world, enlightened parents value both male and female babies and treat them equally. If the family wants to beget a male child, it can be planned. Leaving aside X or Y chromosomes[7], we can say that the gender of the child depends on the husband or male-partner only. The husband should eat well and avoid frequent intercourse. A gap of four or more days between

---

[6]   *Ideal Marriage* by T. H. van de Velde

[7]   Woman has two X chromosomes (XX) and man has one X and one Y chromosomes(XY). When a man's X chromosome is fertilized with a woman's X chromosome, female child is born but when a man's Y chromosome in sperm is fertilized with the woman's egg, male child is born. (Source: Encyclopaedia Britannica DVD)

intercourses may help in begetting a male child. Of course, this should be planned at least 3 months in advance. After the conception is confirmed, there is no limit in the number of intercourses. Women just grow the fertilized egg. Do not be so crazy to have only male babies so that your son may be forced to share a common wife, as happened to Draupadi[8], a princess who married Arjun and his four brothers at the same time and lived happily with them.

It is ideal to have a son and a daughter in a family for proper psychological balancing and natural living. Whatever may be the composition of the children in a family, avoid begetting more than two or three children beyond which it is difficult for parents to provide the necessary physical and psychological needs of the children.

Woman should eat a variety of food including millets, pulses, vegetables, greens, berries and fruits during pregnancy so that she gives birth to a healthy baby.

Marriage implies responsible behaviour towards the spouse, children, and those close to them, particularly their relatives and friends. Treat them with respect.

Above all, the faithfulness of each partner is paramount in living a happy married life. Also, learning to live within one's means is good. Save a little for future uncertainties. Demanding or nagging for something which is very costly or useless may cost the peace of mind of both partners. Happiness comes not by exploiting the weakness of the spouse but by counselling and correcting when the spouse goes wrong.

Mental worries, hunger, infection in the lungs, throat, or nose, etc. may affect marital happiness very badly. Of

---

[8]   Mahabhrata, a Sanskrit epic in India

these, throat infection seriously affects sexual erection in males, but is mostly not diagnosed by individuals. It may be due to tooth-infection also. Mix half - spoonful of salt in a mouthful of warm water and gargle* with that water for about 5 minutes to kill most of the bacteria in the throat. Diabetes and low blood pressure may also cause the problem of sexual arousal for males.

Most of the problems related to reproductive organs may be related to inadequate supply of pure air (oxygen). Female persons who sit for long hours daily for months together may face menstrual irregularity and other problems related to reproductive organs since enough blood will not be supplied to relevant organs. Male persons who sit for long hours daily for months together may face sexual erection problem and infertility related problems. To avoid these problems, take deep breath while standing so that the chest and stomach expands, keep it for about five seconds, or as long as one can hold the breath, and then exhale slowly. This deep breathing exercise can be done for about 15 minutes daily in the morning and evening. Every hour, stand up and walk for about 10 minutes.

Not taking a variety of food including seasonal vegetables and fruits may also cause infertility related problems. Women may be affected by white discharge.

Avoid incestuous marriage -marriage between biologically close relatives. Incest will cause birth defects and congenital diseases to the offsprings.

Avoid polygamy since one cannot fulfil the psychological needs of the spouses and their children, and the psyche of the children would be greatly affected. Many fratricides were committed by the children of kings who had many wives.

Marriage is one of the moments in life when new relationships are introduced or created in the form of spouse, father-in-law, etc. When you cherish the relationship with your spouse, keep in mind that your spouse has already an established relationship with his or her friends, relatives, etc. Ensure that you extend the relationship to accommodate your spouse's friends, relatives, etc. unless any new relationship is not good for the family.

One has to accept the relationship—personal, social, official, etc.—as it is. One cannot accept a relationship with a child ignoring their parents, one cannot accept a friend ignoring his smoking partner, one cannot accept a boss ignoring the irritating personal assistant, etc. Otherwise, the already established relationship with the spouse may become brittle and may cause unnecessary problems in the course of time.

MAN VERSUS WOMAN

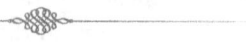

Man cannot exist without woman and vice versa. By god or nature, man and woman play complimentary roles in a family even though most of the roles can be played by both on all times.

For the survival of his progeny, man took upon himself the security of the society and physically strong or risky work like food gathering in the forest.

As time passed, man was the prime gatherer of food and the creator of wealth, and he arrogated to himself the wealth and the power to distribute it. So woman was at the receiving end.

To bring sanctity to his power or authority, male gods were created, and woman was ordained to do according to the wishes of the man or male gods. Even though goddesses were created, accompanying gods as wives, goddesses were subservient to gods, as was in the man-dominated society. Man imprisoned woman psychologically by forcing her to do illogical rituals and humiliating ceremonies, in the name of gods and goddesses.

Even though both man and woman are fallible, man was always given the benefit of doubt while woman was socially ostracised and humiliated.

Men in different societies exploited women in different ways and treated them mostly akin to dignified slaves. They were valued as an object of enjoyment, creators of future progeny or, at most, a kind of valuable property[9] and sometimes bartered[10].

Even though man and woman are interdependent, the arrogance of social authority made man dominate woman in life and subjugate her forever. Since woman had no right over the property of their father, they were always dependent on man for existence. After the death of the husband, to avoid sharing the property with the widow of the deceased, the surviving male members and their relatives encouraged a custom in which the widow was burnt alive in the funeral pyre of her husband.[11] In lawless societies, they are humiliated and treated cruelly since they are forbidden to take up arms.

Enlightened societies gave some respect to women. Due to the shortage of manpower for work since men went to the war front, the world wars forced warring countries in Europe to give employment for women, which was the monopoly of men till then. The financial independence led

---

9   *Mahabharata*, an ancient Sanskrit epic in India tells about Draupadi, a princess who was won in an archery competition by Arjun and married Arjun and four of his brothers. Later, Yudhishthira, the eldest among the five brothers, gambled the common wife in a game of dice and lost her in the game.

10 Francis Parkman, in his travelogue *The Oregon Trail*, tells about a Native American (Red Indian) who offered his pretty daughter in marriage in exchange for the horse of the author. The author declined the offer.

11 A custom called sati was prevalent mostly in Bengal, a part of British India, and the custom was abolished by Lord William Bentinck, a British Governor General of India under the initiative of Ram Mohan Roy, an Indian whose sister-in-law died of sati.

to more rights and an almost equal status in the society in many countries.

Man dominated the society by violence and his monopoly on employment for a long time and continue to sustain it in the name of god and tradition. Woman is weakened by nature during pregnancy and most of her time is spent in bringing up the children, and preparing food for the family which deprives her of essential time to develop her knowledge and skill.

Even in male dominated societies, begetting sons does not guarantee a happy life in a family unless they are brought up properly.

> Akbar, an emperor in ancient India, had three sons. All were addicted to alcohol. Two of them died of heavy drinking. Akbar tried to stop the habit of drinking by his youngest son but he could not succeed. The only surviving son, Prince Salim (who was later called emperor Jahangir), openly rebelled against Akbar to get the throne. Akbar even went with an army to subdue his son but he returned without fighting a war because of the news that Akbar's mother was in death bed[12]. Akbar handed over the kingdom to his son while in death bed.

> A society, in which women do not feel secure, parents feel women are a liability, women cannot share the property of their parents, and women cannot compete with men in the field of their choice, cannot be treated as a civilised society whatever be the luxuries women enjoy.

---

[12] Akbar by Laurence Binyon

PARENTHOOD

Parenthood is an implied responsibility of the parents for the growth of the child as a human being and as a member of the society.

The responsibility assigned to parents by providence or nature looks after the physical and psychological needs of the child, whereas the responsibility assigned by the society looks after the interactive behaviour with members of the society.

If anyone dreams of a bumper harvest without sowing the seeds in time and without watering and tending the plants as required from time to time, then one is living in a dream world. So is the case with a child.

The primary responsibility of a parent is to keep the child as close as possible, both physically and psychologically. Mere feeding does not shape a child. Try to listen to them through their eyes, gestures, words and behaviour and, as far as possible, fulfil their desire if reasonable.

Encourage the children to explore the world around them and guide them to explore the unknown. Take them out as soon as the infants start walking and show them whatever they can see, telling the name of the objects. Feed them whenever they need food-not whenever it is convenient to you. Avoid overfeeding to avoid stomach pain and other problems including obesity.

As soon as they start talking, simply be like a guide to a tourist, explaining simple things in simple words. Never dump facts or words, which they cannot understand. Otherwise, their head may become a dustbin for unwanted words and items. Never think that even after telling many times, your child does not learn. If you feel that by the way you teach, the child should have learnt what you taught, then think about yourself. You would not be what you are, but you might have become a renowned scholar. So have the patience to know the joy of learning new things—if need be, in the hundredth attempt, and if the child feels otherwise, in the thousandth attempt. Never give up. Never shout, or show your angry face, or give any sarcastic comment.

Try to understand the physical and psychological world that the child is in at any time. Try to understand the little friends they like, the little stories they love to hear, the little pets they love to play with, the new world they love to explore with your help, etc.

The child needs your time and attention more than anything else including their favourite toys. Your child needs your constant monitoring, frequent guidance, and occasional help. A small mistake, if not corrected in time, may tempt them to commit blunders.

Parents who try to make a perfect child spoil the child from further learning or exploring. Instead, the child turns out to be a slave waiting for the master's command. So avoid disciplining them too much. Try to counsel them when their mind is receptive, particularly while they are taking food.

Your parents can give a lot of time and wisdom acquired from different experiences to their grand children. So never think that they are a liability. Try to look after them as best as possible. Their knowledge and experience are much more valuable to your child than the food and shelter that you give them.

Never misbehave with your spouse or other family members or never speak a harsh word in the presence of your children. Also, never frown at, or scold, or beat, them without inquiring from them and giving a chance to realise their mistake and to correct themselves in future. Once they grow up, that behaviour will become a normal behaviour, and the grown-up child will be conditioned to behave in the same way with his progeny and the society in later life.

A child, when goes wrong, should be corrected, if need be, forcefully, and frequently counselled when the child is in a receptive mood. When force is used, it should be followed by counselling immediately or later. A child should never feel that whatever he does would be tolerated by the elders. A story told by my teacher in a primary school may be helpful in this respect.

> There was a mother who had a small child. Once, the small child went to a neighbour's house and brought an eyeless needle which was useless. The mother was appreciative about his behaviour. After sometime, he used to steal small items from near-by houses. As he grew up, he started stealing more boldly and brought the items to his house. His mother did not protest or counsel. Once, while stealing, he was caught red-handed and, for escaping, he killed the house-owner. For that, he was sentenced to death. His last wish before dying was to see his mother. As soon as he met his mother, he embraced his

mother and later, he bit his mother's nose.
When the mother started crying, he told her
that had she counselled him while he stole
the eyeless needle, he might not be in this
position.

Different parents bring the children up in different
ways. A psychological scar is more traumatic than a
physical scar and it will haunt the child throughout the
life. With a little more patience, a little more care and a
little more timely response to their needs and queries, can
you bring up your child as a better human being even if
you were denied such little luxuries in your childhood? A
careless parent may spoil the child's mind for ever besides
making the child a liability for the family and the society.

One of the parents can play the role of a
disciplinarian sometimes and the other can
play the role of a benefactor and counsellor
always.

Children are shaped more by the society,
family, and the knowledge and effort of the
individuals than by the hereditary genes. For
healthy genes, give a variety of food. Behave
well with the children, and avoid rude
behaviour or indecent words in the family,
and guide them to find their place in the
society, for they would be the future leaders
of the society.

MOULDING A CHILD

The mind of a child is like clay which can be moulded into any shape, or it can be painted in any colour.

Do you want to make your child as brave as a lion, or do you want your child to be a future child-rearing industry? Do you want your child to hate your neighbour simply because you do not like your neighbour—may be due to genuine reason? Do you want your child to fear the shadow of darkness or the light on truth? Do you like your child to live for the sake of living or to dare death when facing death face-to-face? Do you like your child to fear cockroaches and worms that you loathe to see?

Do you want your child to disown his principles and values simply because you do not agree or simply because the majority is indifferent and not supportive? Do you want your child to disown you simply because you are no longer useful to him?

If your child does not think the way that you think, will you allow him to convince you the way he thinks, or will you force him to follow your way? Within the limit of the norms, will you allow your child to experiment and experience, or will you impose your authority that has been ordained in the name of customs, traditions, and other ceremonies handed over by your forefathers, and about which the child knows nothing?

Yes, you can mould your child in any way you like. But do not expect him to be a scholar after years of training him as a soldier. Do not expect your child to think independently like a philosopher after training her to follow the path shown in the ancient scripture without raising any question. Do not expect your child to look after you in old age when you train your child to observe the ill treatment meted out to your parents who were helpless. Do not bemoan when your child does not listen to you after training him, when he was frail and weak, to obey only your commands without listening to him.

Never expect your child to have an ideal view of life after training him to observe your frequent quarrels with your spouse. Never expect your child to behave decently while you train him by behaving rudely with him.

Children learn more than what you teach. They learn by observing you, your behaviour, your family's behaviour, and the attitude of the society. Yes, you can mould your child the way you like. Your contribution, both direct and indirect, in moulding their future is immense and immeasurable.

But after growing an acacia tree for years together, do not expect apples from it. Also, after growing an apple tree, remember to guard against worms and pests.

Do you have the wisdom to grow the plant the way you dream and the patience to wait for the fruit?

When your child was infirm and weak, have you supported her? When your child was ignorant, have you tried to enlighten her? When your child was lonely, have you given company to him? When your child was sick, have you comforted her or have you kept yourself away, fearing infection?

When the world remembers your child for her contributions, will she remember you for your contribution in bringing her up? Are you matured enough to mould your child as a human being, as a loved member of your family, or as a responsible member of the society? Can you give your time for your child and be a role model to be followed?

A real incident may be useful to all.

> To avoid the horrible heat in summer, a person from South India was walking in the night in a road in Himalayas. He saw a figure hovering before him and it did not move. Fearing, he shouted to give way and it did not move. Then he observed that its legs did not touch the ground. He had heard that ghosts' legs would not touch the ground. Shouting to give way, he ran towards it with a knife and knifed it many times and fainted. When he woke up, he was in hospital surrounded by police who charged him with a murder. Later it turned out that someone has committed suicide by hanging himself in a tree on the road and he had knifed the dead body only[13].

Hence, do not scare children too much in the name of unknown ghosts, gods, satan or any known or unknown persons or objects. Its effects may linger on till one's death.

---

[13] From the book 'Kal Nadaiyil 18,000 miles' (18,000 miles By Walk), a Tamil book by an author(name forgotten) published around 50 years back. It was about his travels by walk, mostly, in India, Ceylon(Srilanka) and a Himalayan country.

CHILD: GROWING UP PHYSICALLY

In the beginning, the only language that an infant knows is crying. Try to understand what the infant is trying to tell. Does the infant feel secure and comfortable by frequent embraces and caressing? Is the infant neat and clean so that there is no itching in the body? Is the napkin dry? Is any fly sitting on the child, or a mosquito biting? Did the mother overfeed, creating a stomach problem? Is the infant lifted frequently so as to release the gas formed in the stomach as flatulence and avoid stomach pain? Are you so audacious so as to wake your child up to show to a friend while it is sleeping? When the child starts crying, do you speak to the child so that the child feels that there is someone to help it? Do you prefer to sleep nearby your child so that you can attend to its needs even though the child is sick and the infection may also spread to you?

Try to adjust to the needs of the child, and do not expect your child to adjust according to your convenience. As the child grows up and as it starts eating other foods besides mother's milk, give food which is easily digestible, preferably, in the form of paste. While feeding milk, mix with 50 per cent water so that the milk is digested easily. Pure milk will produce more waste gas in the stomach, and if not released in time as flatulence, it may cause stomach pain. Check whether the stool is greenish or smelling, which indicates infection. (When we eat food like greens, the stool will be greenish which is normal). Check whether the phlegm is smelling or greenish, which indicates infection.

Persistent crying of infants may be due to the following causes:

i)   lack of sleep or the infant feels sleepy.
ii) hunger or thirst.
iii) stomach pain due to gas in the stomach or physical discomfort like itching in the skin, mosquito bite, wetting the bed etc. and
iv) fear of being alone.

The child may not be able to do things that they normally do like walking, climbing etc when they feel hungry or sleepy or when they have fear or feel any pain.

When teeth start growing, keep the surroundings clean so that the child does not eat anything lying on the ground which may lead to loose motion. Give something like rusk to munch which is hard to bite but easy to digest. Give a variety of food in the form of paste, including seasonal fruits. Minimise giving unseasonal fruits whose effect on the body is different.

The common cold is a common problem which both the child and the parents have to live with. Do not demand an instant cure for the common cold. There is no medicine to kill the 200 and odd viruses causing the common cold. Strong medication to suppress the symptoms may have long-term side effects besides causing irritation to the child. Remove the mucus from the nose gently and frequently with soft dry kerchief. Try to keep the child in an upright position as long as possible to avoid nasal blockage and breathing problems.

Breastfeeding the child as long as possible will keep the child more healthy besides feeling the security of motherhood which will make the child more curious and more intelligent.

When the child is sick, be nearby to console and help. Remember that the child can understand through touch and sound only. So cuddle and embrace, remembering the caution 'handle with care'. Kind words or a lullaby will make the child feel secure thinking that someone is nearby.

The best company to your child is your parents and parents-in-law who can give as much time as the child needs and have the patience and experience to face a child. So do not discard the old people who can give your child the best care for so meagre amount of food and nominal maintenance expenses. Do not dump them in old-age homes.

Never forget to give different kinds of foods in eatable form like juice, food made into a paste, or normal food depending on the age. But never overfeed children. That will deprive the child the joy of learning the surroundings through its senses due to the uneasiness created within the body. You can feed small amounts of food many times, but not too much of food at any time. Tinned baby foods may be given occasionally, but not regularly. It will cause constipation and obesity.

CHILD: CONDITIONING

Most of the children, born to parents of a certain religion or sect following certain traditions, live and die as the followers of the same religion or sect.

The children follow the same rituals which are sacrosanct to the parents. The same rituals had been handed over from generation to generation and practised generation after generation. The vision of the gods, what is good and bad, an ideal life in the society, etc. are imbibed into the minds of the children and are sculptured permanently in the minds and they cannot be erased without causing severe psychological storms and damage to existing structures in the mind. Only a long exposure to other cultures, rituals, etc. will remove the dogma that is sculptured in the mind very slowly.

What was taught during childhood, the manners and behaviours that were followed, and the ideas that were imbibed could not be changed easily during the entire life even when in the midst of another system. So avoid frowning at the child, avoid scolding, avoid deprivation of food, avoid behaving violently, etc. Any conduct which occurs frequently or lasts for a long time becomes a normal behaviour, and it is repeated by the child after the child becomes an adult without the feeling of guilt, even if it is a bad manner.

So bring up your children to observe any system and analyse and accept ideas from any faith even though your ideas are dogmatic.

Before the children, you are the supreme authority which may not be questioned even though lingering doubts are there. So conduct yourself before them so that they will have the faith in your authority and the ultimate authority above you.

Imbibe in the mind of the child that rituals and ceremonies are a means of getting together relatives and friends. If any sanctity is sanctioned on any ritual, tell your children that it is not ordained by any god but for some known or unknown reason associated with the society.

Imbibe in the mind of the child that those who do not do such rituals also live happily in the same way as those who do such rituals.

Be a role model to the child. Conduct yourself before the child the way you expect the child to behave with others. Do not lecture about manners and behaviours too much. After the child observes how you lie to others, never expect the child to be truthful to you. After speaking harsh words or after looking angrily or threateningly for each silly mistake, never expect your child to behave gently with you in the later part of your life. Hereditary traits apart, consciously or unconsciously, the behaviour of parents are imbibed by the children mostly within five years of age.

CHILD: LEARNING AND REARING UP

Children learn more than what you teach. They observe more than what you show. They explore and discover more than what you feel that they would do. In short, they learn more than the dos and don'ts that you teach. They also learn from your conduct.

So learn to behave with them well and learn to behave with others well in the presence of your children. Justifying words may not be able to convince them after they observe your wrong behaviour.

In the beginning, the mother becomes a demigoddess for a child, and later, the father becomes an omnipotent demigod. Will you behave well in your family and in the society, or will your child receive some adverse remarks from his friends about you or from your quarrelling spouse which will adversely affect the ideal image that was in the child's mind?

Do you have the wisdom to understand the children's necessities and fulfil their little expectations? Do you have the patience and time to hear about their little world in which they find pleasure? Are you ready to help them explore the world around them by taking them out frequently? Do you have the mindset to read and tell stories which they would love to hear from you?

Are you satisfied with providing food and toys to your child, or do you find it necessary to find time to be a part of the little world by playing with them? Do you find time to take them out to satisfy their curiosity and explore the unknown world, or are you too busy to spare your valuable time? Sophisticated toys cannot replace you even in their little world. Playing with other children is also a part of learning for them.

Due to instinct or out of curiosity children do a lot of mischief. Do not show your angry face or scold them or beat them. Have the time and patience to convince them. Protect your child from humiliation, ill treatment, harsh words, quarrels, or violent behaviours so that they do not grow up with fear. They are not matured enough to hear a scolding, see a violent scene in a film, see a chicken being killed, see a drunken father squabbling about silly things, see the parents behaving violently or illogically, etc.

CHILD AND EDUCATION

Everyone wants their children to be formally educated and trained for a good life. But we do many things in life which affect their education.

As far as the literary part of education is concerned, the major impact on learning will be made by

i)   your conduct and recognition
ii) sleep and
iii) playing.

If the child dislikes you, whatever you say goes to naught as far as education is concerned. So be persuasive and participative and do not expect immediate results. It may take years together to convince the child or to make the child understand. Never say 'This is good for your future. You must learn.' The child does not know what it means. Appreciate and encourage them to study.

Sleep soothes the mind. Only a calm mind can study and retain it in the memory for a long time. Small children need ten to twelve hours of sleep during the initial stages of schooling and eight to ten hours of sleep in the later part. Without sound sleep, the child can neither be attentive to what the teacher teaches, nor can it study on its own. Also, anything studied without proper sleep is likely to be forgotten within a short time. Irregular sleeping habits affect the studies seriously. If the child has to be woken up frequently or gets up after an alarm sounds, that means the child is not having enough sleep.

During the initial stages, small children cannot concentrate on their books for more than fifteen minutes. So allow them to play to refresh their mind and allow them to start again. Loud reading may help to reinforce learning, particularly in the early stages of learning up to an approximate age of ten.

Children forget quickly. Teach the children and explain to them patiently 10 times, 100 times, or even 1,000 times. Never ask questions. They will come out on their own when you initiate, if they understand. If you do not have the patience to wait for the fruit, stop teaching. Also, stop teaching if the children feel uneasy while you are teaching. An unfit teacher may spoil the mind of the child forever and hence spoil the curiosity to learn even in the future.

Children love to play, and so allow them to play. They are curious to know what is outside their house. Explain what they see and try to correlate what they have studied with what they see.

Tell a lot of stories which they would love to hear—folk tales, fairy tales, and other small stories with animal characters. That will help them to concentrate their mind on hearing and to assimilate them in the mind. This will help them to listen when the teacher teaches. Never try to test them by asking questions or never try to expose their ignorance. They will come forward while narrating the story, when they understand. It may take weeks, sometimes years, to make them understand.

After the child returns from school, give some snacks and ask what he did in the school or what he learned there. That will help him to recollect what he learned in the school and prepare him to be more attentive in the school, for he has to tell the same to his father, mother, or grandparents. Never scold or give any sarcastic comment if they do not know. That will force them to find some excuse to escape from you. Be a student before the child.

While the child studies or does homework, do your work nearby if need be. After the child completes the studies, ask him to explain what he has studied—not as a teacher for testing, but as an inquisitive person to learn more and correct the child if necessary.

Talk a lot to the child—it may be about anything in the house or in the book or outside. That will help the child talk freely and expose his mind—his thinking, fears, expectations, etc. Without free talk, the child may live in a psychological island, forming his own interpretations, ideas, and fears which may be more harmful to him and to the society.

The child never likes the subject which was not understood by him. Try your level best to encourage the child to study. If the child finds it formidable, start from the first stage of schooling, and you will find the wonderful turn for the better in about two to three years. Do not expect miracles immediately, for that will spoil the child psychologically forever.

Never advise your child to concentrate on more than one work at a time. That will distract the mind from doing any work properly, including listening in the class and hence studies.

Advice your child to go to bed before he feels sleepy. That will give ample time to think on what he did on that day including the teaching that he understood, the games he played, etc. You can tell stories while they are lying on the bed before sleeping.

If the child finds it difficult to study, let him study in the same stage or class for one more year. Promoting him to the next stage will further make it difficult to study and weaken the child psychologically, which is the beginning of the end of his studies. Sarcastic comments from the classmates and friends are more demoralizing than the words of teachers and parents. Detention in the right stage helps the child to stand on his own leg.

Girls pick up skills in speaking at a younger age while the boys are slow. But around thirteen years of age, girls' education slows down, most probably due to the loss of essential minerals from the blood while the boys improve slowly. So ensure that the children take a variety of food, particularly all kinds of spices, vegetables, green leafy vegetables, berries and seasonal fruits.

Mere knowledge does not make a person wise or creative or productive. Just like food needs time for digestion, knowledge needs time to be assimilated in the mind and needs associated experiences, experiments, etc. to make it meaningful. Give enough time, to explore and experiment, to the child so that the child understands what is taught instead of dumping information in the mind of the child. Each child needs a time of its own to understand what is taught.

Good health helps the child, to be attentive in the class, and not to miss the class. So keep the child healthy by providing a balanced food – a variety of food including all kinds of vegetables and seasonal fruits.

CHILD: PREPARING FOR LIFE

Just like any animal prepares its baby to face the future and live a life of its own, each parent has a mandate from nature to prepare the children to face the challenges of life. So each one should have a healthy body. Also, each one should have a healthy mind and an acceptable behaviour in the society. Only when we behave well with children even when they do not behave, they will learn to behave well. If necessary, one has to counsel them in the right time. There is no magic to transform them into responsible persons. Parents should initially be a role model for the child. Besides that, the person should have enough knowledge and skill to face the challenges of life. Knowledge does not mean literary knowledge only.

With more and more micro-families and less and less common community centres, the children have lost the joy of non-formal learning about interdependence and living together. Almost complete isolation from the society is harmful to individuals also, for human beings are social animals.

Remember that a child is not a machine to input data and get the desired output. Knowledge has to be imparted in doses which can be digested or assimilated in the mind. That is, knowledge in any subject should be understood before acquiring more knowledge, just like constructing a building brick by brick. Never dump too much information which one cannot understand. It will result in mental problems if tried aggressively.

Based on the acquired knowledge, develop the necessary skills essential for material life. That will help to earn a living for a decent life. Exposure to different situations, places, people, trades, jobs, etc. may help one to hone their skills essential for life. But without enough knowledge, the skills developed may not be of good quality.

While the children acquire necessary knowledge and skill for a comfortable living, teach them that happiness does not depend solely on money and comfort.

CONDITIONING

Conditioning is a process of making a person believe in something or behave in a certain way under certain circumstances through the controlled exploitation of sensual demands or natural urge.

Conditioning may change the behaviour of a person (or any animal) by giving sensual pleasure or pain or by giving a promise of sensual pleasure or fear of pain. The human urge to survive or the fear of death is used by all societies to condition man and woman.

An easy way of conditioning is done by the use of words with the promise of sensual fulfilment or the deprival of sensual needs. Coupled with other sensual needs like hunger, fragrance, comfort, etc., indoctrination with words is an easy form of conditioning.

Each society knows the value of good conduct and behaviour by its members, and no police personnel can go behind each one in the society monitoring the behaviour. So heaven, under the control of the god, was created, and a person with good behaviour was promised perpetual pleasure and comfort in heaven. So, good behaviour of each member of the society was assured with a promise of sensual pleasure in future.

Similarly, hell was created to deter wrong or unwelcome behaviour with a threat of perpetual pain and sufferings.

A promise of a favourite sweet, like chocolate, or the latest electronic gadget may bring some desirable changes in the behaviour of a child. The promise of a ticket to a music orchestra may help parents to make the children to behave, or not to behave, in a certain way.

The fear of prison may deter many from doing illegal things. The fear of reprimand may force a child to keep his room neat and tidy. The promise of a good job and hence a comfortable life may make a person study sincerely. A word of appreciation may make a scientist delve deeply into his work.

Coupled with rituals and ceremonies, conditioning can be symbolically associated with any indoctrination. It is very difficult to come out of such indoctrination. As one participates more and more in rituals and ceremonies, the conditioning is reinforced more and more which results in the refusal to think logically beyond one's conditioned thoughts and behaviour. Most of the beliefs and dogmas related to gods and religions are indoctrinated at a young age through conditioning. Each family and each society finds its own way of conditioning its members by different rituals and ceremonies.

As the rituals and ceremonies become more and more illogical or humiliating, the conditioned person is ready to do anything associated with it—filthy or shameful or violent acts against one's own conscience.

What was fed as nutritious in young age may be taken till later in life even if it was found to be wrong later. A food preferred by oriental people is hardly palatable to an occidental person. A person who was brought up in a village hardly prefers to live his last days in a big city and vice versa.

Training is a form of conditioning. Training conditions a person to operate a machine properly without much thinking, as is the case of typing by a typist.

Proper conditioning of the child, particularly related to manners, etiquette, behaviour, and beliefs, are essential, but illogical or irrational conditioning damages the child psychologically forever. So, it is the way of bringing up the child and the social environment which condition the mind whether one is amenable to reason or extract a pound of flesh[14].

---

[14]   The Merchant of Venice by William Shakespeare: Antonio got loan from Shylock, a money lender on the condition that, if not repaid in time, Antonio should give a pound of flesh from his body. After the due date, when Antonio was ready to give double the amount agreed, Shylock refused to accept it but insisted to take a pound of flesh from the body of Antonio.

OLD AGE

Old age is the time when one has more experience and wisdom to share with others but hardly anyone is interested to listen.

Blessed are those who manage their own affairs and get their needs fulfilled in their old age. But if one has to depend on their family members or relatives for their daily needs and if the family members feel it as a burden, it is really painful. If none looks after the old person, it is pathetic.

It may happen that the children may be too busy to look after the old person or they may be far away. But when one is nearby, if one cannot help the old parents or if one cannot share a few moments in their daily life, it is a pathetic life for the old parents.

But a moment for introspection for the old: when the old parent was a youth, did that youth look after his or her parents as he or she expects from his son or daughter?

In life, we are paid back with the same coin—if we did not look after our old parents, we would get the same treatment as wages for our past labour. A story heard during my school days may help to understand about old age.

> A man was ill-treating his dependent old parents. He started to give stale food in an earthen bowl, which was considered lowly in

the society. After some time, the earthen bowl was missing. He scolded his parents and gave a new one. This was repeated on a few more occasions. At last, the man was angry and scolded the old parents too much. Then his son came and told that he was keeping those earthen bowls safely for his father. When the father becomes old, these earthen bowls will be used for him since the boy would not buy a new earthen bowl if it breaks. The man realized his mistake and treated his father well after that.

Children observe more than what we teach. We get back what we give in life. So never treat old people as a liability.

OLD AGE: WARPED BY TIME

By the laws of nature, man was destined to die fighting for survival and protecting his progeny. But man has protected himself from his predators that, when old and infirm, he has to depend on his progeny and society for help and survival.

In a joint family where there are many members in the family, there will be someone to look after the needs of old people. As the family becomes small and everyone is busy, old people are neglected and, sometimes, humiliated because they have become a liability.

Experiences of old persons, sometimes called wisdom, are useful to everyone in the family, particularly their grandchildren. Hence, it is advisable to look after old parents and treat them with dignity so that they can give their suggestions and opinions in a frank and useful manner.

Also, old persons can have a lot of time to spare. So when you are busy with your work, old parents can become very good companions for their grandchildren. They may tell stories which your children would love to hear or allow the children to explore the neighbourhood under their supervision or give some tips when the infant is weeping for no reason and the like. You cannot have the patience to hear what your child wants to say nor can you spare so much time. So try to keep your parents with you when they are old and look after them to the extent possible.

A FEW WORDS FOR OLD PEOPLE

Old age is an inevitable experience of life. Only the luckiest will die a peaceful life.

Old people have more experience, and hence, they should have more wisdom and patience. So they should conduct themselves with grace and treat the young and the children with dignity. They should have the mental maturity of never misbehaving with children and be trustworthy.

Due to damaged teeth, old people may not be able to eat a variety of food. Hence, diseases may affect in old age, and so, medical expenses may rise. So while young, people should have saved a little bit when they earned a lot. Of course, at a time when we are busy with our immediate needs and are more inclined to enjoying life, it is difficult to foresee or think such a possibility at a young age.

Infants digest 100 per cent milk but old people cannot digest milk fully. Minimise milk in the food. If taken, add more than 50 per cent water, for easy digestion.

As one becomes older and older, the physical faculties become less and less sharp. So the physical needs should be less and less. So never compete for more privileges when you are old. Plum resources should go to the breadwinners and the growing children.

When your children become young, they may not have time to spend with you. They have to work for more money. They have to explore the world and acquire new experiences. They have to enjoy life with spouse, children, friends, etc. So never jostle for their time in your life. Any interference in their life will be treated as an encroachment of their rights by an enemy.

Old people cannot run with the time of the young, and if they try, only a sense of dragging will be felt. Have the maturity of mind to find your own space and own time which are, of course, standing still. Keep yourself busy by doing some useful work for your children and grandchildren by reading books, reinventing your hobby, doing something useful to the society, etc.

But when your children go wrong, never hesitate to show the right direction, whether they like it or not or whether they follow your advice or not. They may change later, after some new experiences.

As long as old parents are useful to their son or daughter, they can stay with their son or daughter. As soon as they are less useful, it is better for the old parents to stay separately to avoid a feeling that they are a liability. The closeness of like minds causes friction and heat sometimes, whereas the separation of even incompatible minds creates a sense of calm in the mind of both the young and the old. But dependent living always brings a sense of liability.

Medical care is a big business and not a service in most of the places. So never allow treating your disease by your children, which will make them liable to work for their entire life. Is the existence of a diseased old man really crucial for a happy life in the family, or will he survive just like a dead wood in a tree? Can the old man contribute something worthwhile for the family or the society? Should an old man become a liability for his children even after his death?

Old people cough too much due to infected throat which may be due to infected teeth or lungs. Gargle* with warm salt-water weekly to avoid this and clean the mouth with pure water after gargling. On some bacteria in the throat and respiratory tract, gargling may not work. Inhale steam from hot water through the mouth to kill them. Never eat hot food or hot drinks to kill the bacteria. It may damage your teeth or the food pipe (oesophagus). Avoid hot dry air also to soothe the throat.

Our nerves die every day, and they cannot be regenerated. So our sensual functions cannot function optimally forever. So never dream of living forever. A ripe fruit has to leave the tree for an unknown destination and an unpredictable future. A useless old leaf has to fall down to give space for a fresh new leaf in a tree. There is no evergreen life or everlasting life. Dream for a death with less pain for you and less burden to your near and dear ones.

When your children were weak and needed constant monitoring and help, did you ever volunteer to do the work for the child and relieve your spouse for some time, or did you pretend that you were too busy to spare any time for the child? When you are old and infirm, do you expect your children to help you? When your child was having the common cold or simple diseases, did you cuddle your child with kind words or did you keep yourself away, fearing infection? When you are sick, do you expect that your child would attend to your needs? Throwing away the toys, when the child longed for your company, did you manage politely or did you command to obey your order?

When you are lonely and depressed, do you expect that your child would support you? Do you want special rules and privileges for you, but not for your child? Recollecting the past may bring down the expectation and calm the mind.

Have a clear conscience and be ready to face death at its face like Socrates[15] rather than clinging to life like a dead wood in a tree. But, when one is physically frail and mentally weak, can one face death boldly and be ready to fathom the mysteries of the shadows of life?

---

[15]   Socrates, an ancient Greek philosopher was charged that he spoiled the minds of the youth and was condemned to death because of his views. His friends insisted that he should escape to some other city state, but Socrates preferred to die, taking poison in his city state, Athens.

FATE

The cause and effect of our actions percolates to others—family, friends, neighbours, society, etc. That is, the effect of one's thoughts and actions are felt by others. A drunken driver injures a few people in an accident. A philanthropist changes the future of so many orphans. There are incidents in life when one feels that one should not have run after money madly; one should not have run after beauty madly; one should not have harassed people; one should have helped an accident victim; one should have given more time for the children; one should not have used the power for personal gratification; one should have invested the savings in certain company; one should not have trusted a person; one should not have done the way a work was done; etc. Sometimes, an unknown person or some unrelated thing changes our course in life in spite of the minute execution of our plan. Let us call it fate.

Death is an inevitable part of life. What about the events between birth and death? Are they predetermined by god?

If both tiger and deer are created by god, then fate is the only option for human beings because god, the Creator, has to feed both the hungry tiger and the hungry deer. If nature has created the tiger and deer during the course of evolution, then it has to keep itself in balance. If one is fighting the pangs of hunger, the other is struggling for survival. Will one get the next meal? Will the other survive death? None knows for sure till time goes by a few minutes into the future.

A carefully prepared plan fails due to some unknown factor. Who thought that Napoleon Bonaparte[16] would have stomach ache just before the Battle of Waterloo? Similarly, an accidental work may bring out some wonderful products. Sir Alexander Fleming's[17] discovery of penicillin was based on an accidental observation.

What will happen in the next moment in the future is not known. If everything is predetermined by god as fate, then why should one take responsibility for the mistakes done? Is there any purpose of living, or is there no purpose except living anyhow?

Human beings, as members of the society, are bound by the laws of the land and the unwritten laws of the society in the form of social etiquette. The punishment handed over for criminal activities and the rewards given for responsible work are due to the social norms followed in the society. But who is responsible for a lavish lifestyle by one person and a painful and pathetic life for another person? Is it because of god or fate? If so, is god so indifferent or cruel that one shudders to think? Was that cruel event for the reminiscence of the notorious past

---

[16]   Napoleon Bonaparte was a French General and emperor who could not start his battle in time due to stomach ache. Also, due to his communication not reaching the right person in time and other strategic factors, he lost the battle to British General Arthur Wellesley in a place near Waterloo.

[17]   Sir Alexander Fleming, while working on influenza, observed that a plate containing waste (mould) destroyed bacteria, and that resulted in the discovery of penicillin, an antibiotic.

conduct of the parents? Of course, 'if one harms others in the forenoon, then that harm comes back automatically in the afternoon.'[18] When we do not get back for our omissions and commissions in our life, the effect of a deed or misdeed is passed on to our progeny to be experienced during our lifetimes or after death. Or was a cruel event in our life the culmination of bitter thoughts or envy in our mind? Is there any other reason? None knows.

One's effort gives some positive return even if luck or fate, a form of providential interference, also plays its part in life sometimes. But without effort, there is no luck. Even if fate is inevitable, the effort to succeed will surely give some positive experience useful for the future. So believe in yourself and start working with hope for a better future.

A rocket with a 100 per cent chance for success fails due to some unknown reason while a casual plan succeeds because of a change in government policy. So fate and luck play a part in our life when we make an effort to succeed even if we do not know the secret behind it.

Just like any animal, humans are born selfish with an urge to survive. So each one's behaviour depends mostly on selfishness and emotion rather than reason and logic. So our life is a logical sequence not only of events and thoughts but also of incomprehensible random events and thoughts. So life is a mixture of a known effort and an unknown fate.

> A good and reasonable man in a town
> never harmed anyone. He has two sons.
> Both are good and highly educated. Each one
> wanted that the other should do well. But,

---

[18]   Thirukkural: An ancient book in Tamil, a South Indian language.

after some time, on some flimsy grounds, both started quarrelling just like enemies. The good man was excommunicated by a small society because of an effort by a dishonest man. The good man's past revealed that he and his elder brother used to fight (around 30 years before these incidents) on flimsy grounds. Using his influence, the good man used to excommunicate his brother based on small incidents. The good man witnessed similar incidents in his life later.

There was one teacher who never bothered to go to the class or to teach the students. He had seven sons. In that part of India, sons were preferred, for they would bring brides with a lot of dowry during their marriage. The more they studied, the more would be the dowry. But, except one who passed the school examination with great difficulty, six of them were dropouts from the school.

Mahabharata, a Sanskrit epic in India, narrates a story in which Kunti, wife of King Pandu, begot four sons from four different demigods. Madri, Pandu's second wife begot twins from another demigod(twins). The eldest son of Kunti was born before marriage and was abandoned. The rest lived with Kunti. Later in life, the five persons married a single Princess Draupadi and lived most of their life with her only.

So, we get back what we give, of course, in different forms. But, why should one suffer the consequences of someone else's mistakes?

EFFORT AND LUCK

The dreams of a man may take him to unknown heights or untold miseries. But what is ordained by god or nature for a person may not be that person's dream. The urge to succeed is innate, but success is rarely achieved by everyone every time. Mere effort does not guarantee success, but a little bit of luck is also needed in terms of place, person, resources, time, etc. A perfect plan may fail sometimes.

Whatever may be the reason for the failure of one's dream, effort and perseverance never go waste. It rewards with rich experience, acquaintance with right people, knowledge of technical expertise, etc.

A person who believes only in luck is doomed to fail in most of the aspects in life, and neither god nor man can help those idle persons who believe in, and wait for, luck to do their work. In general, there is no luck without effort even though there are isolated cases of luck showering its blessings on idle hands.

The progress made by mankind is attributed to those who dared and persevered while others lived in comfort or feared to perform.

LUCK AND CATASTROPHE

In life, there are always incidents which bring a fortune of plenty or a misfortune of greater effect.

In everyone's normal life, there are seasons of plenty, of withering, and of scarcity in a random order. But only a few may be lucky enough to get the plenty given by fortune without much effort. On the other hand, a few unfortunates may face a catastrophe of immeasurable magnitude by losing everything in spite of every effort to keep everything in order. As in a storm or earthquake, a treasure earned in a lifetime may be destroyed in seconds.

Luck may not pay in plenty many times, but sometimes, catastrophes may not take away everything, if there is a constant effort to persist and succeed.

Since luck and catastrophe are only chances and there is no guarantee for their occurrence, believing only in luck may land one nowhere. In search of luck, people buy lotteries, gamble the hard-earned money, go in search of casinos, etc. Luck is a random phenomenon, and hence, never go in search of luck unless it comes to you. Also, money got through luck is easy money, and it disappears with the speed with which it came unless luck is supplemented with hard work.

In spite of the catastrophe that befell on us, we never felt that we are lucky to be born without physical or mental defects; we never felt that we are born to compassionate parents; we never thought that we have a lovely child; we never thought that we are lucky to earn more than our requirements; we never thought that we are lucky not to be affected by any serious life-threatening diseases; we never thought that we are lucky in living in a society which gives freedom of thought and expression; etc.

None is endowed with everything in life. With what we are lucky to have in life, let us enrich life more by our effort without waiting for luck to do the work for us. If catastrophe befalls, let us pray and hope that we should be able to manage, if necessary, with the help of compassionate helping hands.

THE LUCKIEST

We are one of the luckiest in this world. We are lucky to be without hunger and without worry about our next meal. We are lucky to be born without defects even though some are born handicapped. Even though birth is not chosen by us and we are not born to rich parents, we are lucky to have understanding parents though some children fear their father or mother with silence written on their faces. We are lucky to live without serious ailments even though some live with serious health problems. We are lucky to have a supportive family in spite of our failure in our effort to succeed. We are lucky to live in a sociable society even though it is far away from the city.

We are lucky to have good teachers who endowed us with necessary skills to survive in this world and necessary thoughts to think about life. We are lucky to have a doctor who diagnoses the disease with symptoms and prescribes only essential medicines and advices how to prevent the disease in the future. We are lucky to have a friend who supported us morally while we were in distress.

We are lucky to have a Good Samaritan who helped us after an accident and sent us to a hospital. We are lucky to be born in a country where laws do not ill-treat us simply because of our birth, gender, race, colour, beliefs, etc. We are lucky to have social institutions which protect us from thugs and antisocial elements. We are lucky to be in a society where we can protest against the government itself which governs us. We are lucky to be born as a human being with proper shelter and enough brain to protect ourselves from other animals. We are lucky to live here where no animal has attacked us even though we occupy their habitat.

One is lucky to be endowed with beauty, another is endowed with money and wealth, someone else is blessed with a child while her neighbour is understanding and cooperative, etc.

Do we see the unlucky ones or the unfortunate ones with sympathy or empathy? Shall we ever extend our helping hand to the unfortunate ones when they need our help?

GOD

God is a belief and the belief in god gives hope in life. For a person who is helpless, god is the only hope. Without hope, there will be anarchy in society.

Within the broad parameters of life in nature like birth and death, uncertainties and the unpredictability of events in life with serious consequences made man to think that there is someone above who controls nature. Who is he or who is she or what is that?

In a predominantly male-dominated society, man perceived god in his own image. Gods liked the sweets that he liked. Gods disliked the bitter things that he did not prefer to take. Gods wanted a man to behave as he expected others in the society to behave with him. Gods hated those whom he hated.

Is god alone? Can god survive without a female companion? So goddesses were created. The type of behaviour that is expected from the members of the society on different occasions was imposed on society as that ordained by gods and goddesses.

What was going on in the name of god became so rigid that it started harming the fabric of society. Great thinkers and reformers tried to free the society from the clutches of outmoded rules and traditions going on in the name of god. Since the same gods cannot change the rules that they have ordained, the social reformers talked on the authority of a different god to impose a new set of modified rules and regulations.

As time passed, the purpose, for which the reformers and thinkers fought, was ignored, and the followers made the reformers as gods or representatives of gods. The new rules became dogmas. Once that was done, what were left were a few rituals and ceremonies to show others in the society that they are the faithful followers of their gods.

Why does man fight and die for his gods and goddesses? When a god's supremacy is accepted, the vast empire of the faithful is a source of power for a few, a source of income for many, and a source of moral supremacy over others who are unfaithful. So for the supremacy to be maintained, they have to fight the infidels and increase the number of the faithful. Even those who accept a god differ in their perception about that god and form splinter groups. They start fighting to establish their group's supremacy.

Strangely enough, man fights and dies for his gods, but no god ever died for his faithful followers and devotees.

In the history of human beings, god-men and self-styled agents of god formed a network that made a big business in the name of their gods and goddesses.

If the offerings offered to god can bring blessings, wealth, and other necessities of life, one is having in mind a degraded and deformed god. Can the god, the owner of all things in the world, be fooled by a few offerings so that the devotees get the best things in life in return? For such people, faith in god is just a bargain for a comfortable material life.

What about the real god or goddess? How does he or she look like? Does god want anything from humans? Why does god not intervene to do things the way the god wants? Where is the god? Since man's evolution into an intelligent human being is ordained by god, why did he allow man and woman to discover a few laws of nature which the god set in the beginning? Why good people suffer while the bad or the non-believers of the god enjoy life?

If the answers to the above questions are known, the world would become uniform—smooth and polished in all respects to abide by the will of the god. Even a lion may fast unto death rather than eating venison to comply with the laws of god and defy the laws of nature!

GOD: BELIEF AND HOPE

The history of mankind has shown clearly one thing—the nature of god or the image of god or goddess depends on the belief and values cherished by the society. Man has created god in his own image. That is, god is the embodiment of the society's beliefs and hopes. Under the clutches of immoral priests, even gods became immoral in some societies!

Time played a major role in enlightening the society and forced to change the values that the society cherished for long. The gods that evolved, after the old gods and goddesses were sidelined, were more humane or were need-based to safeguard the changed values and customs.

As Leo Tolstoy has observed, all the religions have outlived the purpose for which they were created. The original values and beliefs were forgotten and only rituals survived, symbolic of the cherished values which are observed in obeisance and supplication in the name of god and religion.

The god which has created men and women also set some rules and customs to bind them in a society. So religion, with all its rituals and ceremonies, has become an unwritten statute to be followed, and god has become its governor monitoring its followers.

A person who travels and observes the world finds that what his god despises is done by a man in another corner of the world with the approval of that man's god. Strange as it is to the traveller, why does his god allow such sin to be done? Since human beings are conditioned by the society directly and indirectly with the values cherished by it in the childhood itself, the statute of the new gods and goddesses may be difficult to comprehend unless it is perceived with the mindset of a new society.

For a man with a conscience, god is observing all for the final reward, whereas for a scoundrel, there are easy ways for salvation, particularly through some rituals like ablutions, offerings, flattery in the form of prayer, rituals, etc.

God's laws were transgressed by men frequently with impunity, and men's laws, defined in the name of god, were transgressed by god frequently to the bewilderment of the god-men and self-styled agents of god who speak in the name of god.

From the beginning of the world, man has considered god as a saviour, as a panacea for his illness, or as a donor giving wealth and comfort. Man was so selfish that he offered a small portion of what he liked to demand a big share from his god. Man believes and hopes that god would give what he prayed for.

For a man who lost hope, god is the only hope left. So, god is an invisible psychological force protecting society against anarchy and reinvigorating a person's energy to look for alternatives.

Any society survives with the belief in the god and the hope it provides, as it happened from the beginning of life. Of course, no other reason is available except the will of god to explain the vagaries of life.

GOD VERSUS SATAN

If god has created the deer, then who has created the lion which kills it? If god has created comfort and happiness, then who causes misery and pain? Why can god not give perpetual victory, happiness, or comfort? Is there an equally invincible Satan, an evil spirit challenging god perpetually—going down sometimes and rising up on another time, but never defeated permanently?

If one sees the contours of life of most of the human beings, one can easily conclude that one is paid back with the same coin—a good deed with a good deed. One's deeds may be paid back in the form of health, wealth, peace of mind, etc. In spite of the seasonal variations in life which is at different levels for each person, one begets what one deserves by his work and thought. The rewards may be positive or negative, and it may be physical or psychological.

So based on one's deeds or thoughts in a fluid social environment, one can visualize the impact on the body, mind, and the neighbourhood within whose boundary the person's influence exists.

Without the twelve labours of Hercules[19], Hercules cannot be a hero. So god and Satan form a unique combination just like the north and south poles of a magnet or day and night of a day or the head and, its obverse, tail of a coin which does not exist in isolation.

So god and Satan are indistinguishable—that is, both are of the same entity. God cannot exist in isolation.

---

[19]   Greek mythology: Heracles, popularly known by his Roman name Hercules, worked under the king of Mycenae to redeem his sin. He was told to do twelve difficult tasks which included killing a lion which could not be killed by any weapon, cleaning the Augean staples, bringing the golden apples of the Hesperides, and bringing the three-headed dog guarding the world of the dead.

GOD VERSUS GOD

In the name of god, men were fighting among themselves to establish the supremacy of their gods and goddesses, and innumerable men had lost their lives. But it has not dawned on men that no god has ever died for his men and only men die for their gods.

Does the all-powerful Almighty not want its men to win a war against the worshippers of other gods? Why do the people of another religion with a different god to worship, different rituals to do, and different moral values to follow survive? How can people of a different faith win a war against the faithful?

From time immemorial, there were people who exploited the name of god as a rallying point for political and social purposes. To enhance their political and social leverage, a few powerful or influential persons made their subjects fight wars in the name of gods.

People were also happy to fight for their gods since they could enjoy the wealth of the defeated. But what about those who died for their gods? The dead of both the winners and the losers were promised heaven, a place for perpetual comfort and enjoyment. If both winners and losers go to heaven, will they find bliss there or will they fight for their gods there also? Divinity and sacredness were attached with wars in the name of god so that none would run away in case of danger from an enemy.

All gods survived with their surviving devotees— men who won in the name of their gods or men who lost because of their fate. While one was celebrating the victory of one's god, the others were bitter and raging to avenge their defeat, not for the defeat of their god.

In each society, when there is a conflict with selfishness or wisdom, it is mostly the selfishness which wins. So fighting in the name of gods is inevitable.

With each new god, there is a new group of people who claims the privilege of speaking, and doing, in the name of the new god. So, the priests of old gods find it hard to lose the privileges associated with their gods and ensure that the new gods and their new set of priestly-class are destroyed and humiliated. So men, who believed in the gods which speak only through their priests, were ready to wage war against the unfaithfuls and infidels.

When god, religion, the scriptures, and the associated rituals do not withstand the scrutiny of reason due to changed times, there is always a conflict of interest between god's man and men's gods.

GOD AND GOD-MEN

If god or nature has created man, woman, and the world, man has created gods and goddesses with the characters and values of his own. With people in the society being conditioned for good behaviour in the name of gods and goddesses, there was a need to look after the needs of gods and goddesses and creating a good image for them by appointing a full-time caretaker for them.

In the course of time, the caretakers became agents of gods, and these god-men started talking in the name of gods. As time passed, the words of the god-men became the words of gods and goddesses. So the words of the god-men should be obeyed just like the order of the king. Of course, they were very careful in pleasing the powerful kings and the privileged.

Man being selfish, god-man also started exploiting god for his own ends, particularly when the devotees had full faith that god can be approached only through a god-man, the agent of god.

As the number of devotees increased, the name of god became synonymous with business, and special interest groups were established in the name of god. Since god is a bond interconnecting each member of the society, the god-man can manipulate as per his wishes or as per the wishes of special interest groups.

No person can represent another person forever since one's will and perception change in the course of time due to various reasons including new facts and experiences. If anyone claims to represent god or speak in the name of god in absolute terms, remember that behind the mask of god, there is something brewing against god's will in his mind. No god has authorized anyone to speak or act in its name. Only the ignorant or extremely selfish man speaks in the name of god's will. As long as the words of god-man do not withstand the ordeal by conscience or reason, never believe the words of any god-man fully.

GOD: EXISTENCE

The existence of god is debated from time immemorial, and its existence is told in terms of hypotheses and surmises based on human experiences by common men, philosophers, etc.

For a person whose needs are satisfied, the existence or non-existence of god is immaterial.

But is there any god or are there gods which are indifferent to the destruction, vices, diseases, etc. which exist in this world? If god exists, why do these vices and diseases survive?

In spite of the random thoughts and behaviour of each human being, if one sees one's life in conjunction with the parents' life, one can conclude an orderliness in life. That is, one is paid back with the same coin—a good coin with a good coin and a fake coin with a fake coin.

The coin that one gets back may be in the form of good and understanding children, money or comfort, health, diseases, indifferent parent or society, etc. A person, who did not look after his old parents, finds himself in the same position later. A man, who fought for more share of his property from his family members, finds his children fighting for unequal share. A person, who swindled money from his business partner, finds that his health has gone down before comprehending what went wrong. A person who helps others finds that his children are helped by

Good Samaritans. Ask your parents about the strange things that are happening to you even though you are good. It may be for your parents to witness and to redeem for their past conduct or it may be for a bitter thought in your mind.

So beyond the natural laws of science, there is something spiritual or supernatural which cannot be understood or predicted that channels one's life. One can call it god. But never shackle its hands and legs with unbreakable rules in scriptures, wasteful rituals, and costly ceremonies. Never claim the ownership of god in exchange of your prayers, offerings, rituals, conduct etc. Never try to remove from its kind heart your bitter enemies simply because they are your enemies.

GOD: THE INFINITY

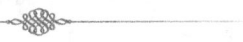

When one sees a few things, one may have a feeling of understanding something, but when one sees infinitely many things, the effect on the mind may be puzzling and strange. Can one comprehend what is infinite, as is said about the omnipresent, omnipotent, or omniscient god?

Let us talk about some infinite matter.

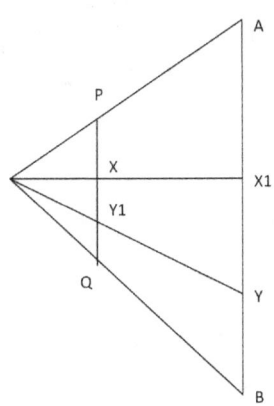

If PQ has a length of 1 centimetre (cm) and AB has a length of 10 kilometre (km), by drawing appropriate lines, one can associate each point X in PQ with exactly one point X1 in AB and vice versa.

That is, there are exactly the same number of points in 1 cm (PQ) as in 10 km (AB).

Similarly, one can prove that there are as many points in a segment with a length of 1 cm as in a segment with a length of thousands of kilometres.

Can one believe this?

If we can believe this, can we believe that a bent curve or a zigzag curve has the same number of points as that of a 1 cm, or 1000 km, segment?

Similarly, since light travels in a straight line, there are exactly the same number of points in a 35 mm film as in a big screen where it is projected. In a never-ending straight line, every point is the centre of the line since there are equal number of points on both sides of that point!

In the structure of a small invisible atom, the movement of electrons and protons is almost similar to the macro planetary solar system with planets moving around the sun!

Of course, when we encounter infinity, there is something incomprehensible or which is beyond simple logic or which can be interpreted in different ways. Most people believe that god is omnipotent, omniscient, infinite, etc. Can we believe this? If we can believe this, can we say there is a projection of god, the Infinite, on our soul or mind in the form of conscience? If so, is there a Satan, the obverse side of god, in our mind in the form of extreme selfishness or greediness?

When extreme selfishness or greediness grows in our mind more and more, there is less and less space for kindness or empathy and vice versa. Whether each one's heart is the abode of god or that of Satan depends on the extent of projection of god, the infinite on the mind in the form of conscience, or of the projection of Satan, the infinite on the mind in the form of extreme selfishness.

That is, those without conscience can never find the god either in idols or in scriptures or anywhere else.

When god resides in your heart, why do you search god outside through brokers and agents who suck the blood of the society and spoil the society by injecting poison in the minds, just like mosquitoes? Be humane and reasonable.

RELIGION

Every person is free as an individual, but as a member of the society, one is bound by implicit, and explicit, rules and traditions of the society. For a smooth life in society, each member of the society has to observe certain common code of conduct which was implemented under the authority of god. Thus, religion was born. Rituals and ceremonies were associated with certain codes of conduct like taking a bath before going to church or temple to emphasize cleanliness, kneeling down before god as a show of obedience, etc.

What are civic laws and penal codes for modern society, it was religion and rituals for our ancestors. The dos and don'ts were compiled. What is thought to be good for the society should be followed, and what is bad should be avoided. Since the rules were implemented in the name of god, not following the good rules or doing the forbidden things invoked the wrath of the god. More than the wrath of the god, excommunication from the society also deterred the members of the society to follow the set of rules of the religion since cooperative living in a society is essential for the survival of any individual.

The rules were framed in the beginning, keeping in mind the condition of the society, and a tradition was established. As time changed, the society changed. The rules and traditions became outmoded. But when the rules became so rigid that the society cannot follow, new religions or different sects of the same religion owing allegiance to the same god were born.

Even then, people belonging to a religion were identified by the rituals and ceremonies rather than the faith in the religion or god. Of course, faith is invisible, but rituals are palpable.

FESTIVALS

For keeping a society in a closely knit unit, periodic rejuvenation of the bonds that shaped the society are essential. For that purpose, festivities and celebrations were organized for the gods and goddesses.

The festivals gave the members of the society the necessary break from the routine work and the required enjoyment with a bountiful of tasty food.

To make the festivals more enjoyable, the festivities were organized after the harvesting season, and the seasonal food was offered to god with thanks for the harvest and a prayer for a good harvest next year.

Some other festivals were organized keeping in mind the seasonal changes and the position of the sun and moon.

Since festivals were organized in the name of god, the locality should be cleaned, the houses should be whitewashed, and the people should be neat and clean. In modern parlance, it is a type of annual inspection with the omnipresent god as inspector. Since god would visit the house and give blessings, houses were cleaned, useless items were discarded, and the rest of the items were rearranged for a better use or a better aesthetic look.

For most of the members of the society, festivals give the necessary relief and rest after a period of monotonous and hard work. So the poor in the society prefer to borrow money and enjoy the fun in life rather than living a debt-free life and foregoing the good things in life. Of course, festivals are tools for social get-together.

HEAVEN AND HELL

Heaven and hell are intertwined concepts which were brought into the minds of human beings by great thinkers and social reformers to bring some accountability to what people do. Who does not want comfort and enjoyment in life? In a world with pain, fear, and difficulties, the dream of a reward for a good work, which appears to be improbable in this world, is really wonderful. So heaven was promised for good and faithful followers of god after death.

In an open society in which none can be monitored forever, the concept of heaven and hell was an innovation which brought some accountability in life, particularly to those who do not bother about their conscience. It helped in conditioning the mind in doing good things approved by the society without being monitored. By nature, man is selfish, but if most of the people in the society do not do socially acceptable things in life, the society can hardly survive.

If people failed to do good things or if they do bad things in life, then as everyone observes, they may not be punished in this world, but punishment after death in hell is inevitable. This deterred people from doing things not approved by the society, particularly when there is a god monitoring all our activities.

EPHEMERAL HEAVEN

Where are hell and heaven? When man believed that the earth was flat, heaven was in the sky and hell was underground. Since anyone is paid back with the same coin—a good coin with good coin and a counterfeit coin with counterfeit coin—heaven and hell cannot exist except in this real world.

A person is in heaven or hell according to the physical or psychological environment that one creates. For a person in hell, the physical environment may be good, but mentally, that person may be in a conflagration which cannot be extinguished. A person with a few material things may be more happy and contented than the rich and powerful.

Heaven and hell cannot be created in one day, but it is formed according to the values that are imbibed throughout the life and the conscience that one possesses.

Do not waste your time and energy in search of heaven. Try to make a heaven physically and psychologically in which you can enrich your life and be at peace.

Anything which lasts forever cannot be a heaven. Anything which lasts cannot be pleasing and comfortable.

The comforts that one loves to live with, the sweets that one loves to eat, the music that one loves to hear, the delicious food that one likes to eat, the circle of friends that one likes to have, the beautiful dreamworld of cinema that one loves to see, etc., when continued beyond a certain level, become boring and unpleasant. As time passes, what looked like heaven loses its charm slowly. When the environment of heaven is prolonged more, the gates of hell start opening.

PRAYER AS HOPE

If god is a belief, then prayer is a hope. A person without hope loses confidence in himself and does not trust the society. Such a person can inflict harm to oneself or to the society. So wise forefathers dangled the magic carrot of hope before the eyes of everyone so that life moves on till the natural end.

Prayer is a form of sedative which calms the turbulent mind and helps to tolerate extreme physical and mental conditions. Hoping for a better situation or favourable condition, each person prays to god.

Prayer imbibes two things—one is that god is omnipotent, and the second is that god is benevolent. Both help to have faith in god and the society which cherishes that god. For a helpless or desperate person, hope is the only way to survive, and prayer gives the necessary hope.

Since prayer alone cannot get things done, one's knowledge, effort, and belief play important roles in accomplishing one's prayer.

There are many occasions in life which are shaped by innumerable constraints and invisible forces. Their permutations and the probable outcomes are innumerable that a rational thinking may lead to mental fatigue or tension. During those times, when everything is beyond one's control or comprehension, it is better to pray with hope rather than worry and spoil mental peace.

PRAYER AS EXPECTATION

Prayer is a reiteration of hope, and each prayer has a lingering faith and expectation for a better future.

In life, what one can change is limited while what comes as the future is unpredictable, and it may turn out to be beyond one's control. So what one dreams of in real life is turned into a prayer.

What type of prayer does one like to pray to one's gods and goddesses? Is it like a bargain, for example, trading spices for food?

Is it a prayer that offers sweets and delicacies to one's gods and goddesses to be taken back and eaten by the very same person who offered it?

Is it a prayer that emanates from the inner feelings of the heart that stood the test of conscience?

Is it a prayer that offers to share a small value of a booty to gods and goddesses?

Will one's prayer stand on a moral plane or a selfish plane? Do your gods and goddesses stand in the same plane where you are standing and make a deal with you, or do you feel that they are in a higher plane, monitoring and guiding you? Are your gods so selfish that they accept your prayers, sweets, and other offerings which you offer as bait?

Have faith in yourself and in your prayer and strive to achieve it. Do not be so selfish as to think that your gods and goddesses are as selfish as you are.

A PRAYER (PERSONAL)

O god! Give me the ability to understand you as you are instead of interpreting you as I think you should be and also the mental strength to accept you as you are.

O god! Let me not belittle you by getting my demands fulfilled by enticing you with flattery in the form of prayer and with offerings in the form of sweets, food, etc. O god! Let me not think that I can befool you by performing a few strange rituals liked by you in exchange for a list of demands of my liking.

O god! Kindly enlighten me so that I am not under any illusion that I am your favoured devotee simply because I am reading the scriptures daily and you would behove an abundance of material benefits to me.

O god! If you have created the lion and the deer, when will you be the saviour of the deer and when will you feed the lion? O omnipotent god! If you have created a faithful like me together with a heretic as a neighbour, let me not have a shred of thought that I am pleasing you by fighting to death with that unfaithful neighbour-just another of your creation. Give me the strength of mind to accept my neighbour as created by you and, as far as possible, coexist within our own boundaries of mind. Let me not claim that the domain of my god in my mind does not contain the domain of that small god in the infidel's mind and so I should subjugate that infidel physically since you are incapable of doing it psychologically by converting him to my fold. Above all, due to business rivalry, due to his majestic and decent behaviour, due to my ill-will to loot some of his property, due to my incapability to compete with him fairly, etc., O god, let me not wait for an opportunity for a communal flare up in your name to kill my neighbour.

O omniscient god! Let me not think that you are incapable of understanding my mind and I am obliged to show my faithfulness only by external features like hair, beard, specific dress, external symbols in the forehead, wearing a talisman, etc.

O god, the infinite! Let me have the wisdom not to mould you as an idol or bind you into a scripture and claim that I know your thoughts and needs. Let me not bind you in the words of scriptures or measure you with special shapes and confine you with strange rituals.

O god! Give me the courage to think that you have not appointed any agent or middleman to represent you in this world and their words are not as sacrosanct as your commandments. Let me not feed the self-styled agents of god so as to outgrow their size and speak on your behalf. Give me the wisdom to think that the social institutions that speak in your name are nothing but, for society, established by the society to streamline the thinking and the course of the society.

O god! Let me not humiliate women or a section of the society as your unimportant or defective creations and impose reparations in the form of harsh and unnatural rituals that they should do or follow unreasonable rules as ordained in your name.

O god! Let me have the courage to accept a person as your perfect creation if one acts with a clear conscience, whatever idols one uses to represent you, whatever words one uses to describe you, and whatever scriptures one claims to follow.

O omnipotent god! Let me not blame the pain and sufferings in this world on Satan or someone else whom you cannot overpower but is a part of life to mould my path.

O god! Give me the maturity of mind not to blame others for my mistakes or claim credit for other's works.

O god! Guide me in this life to live a full life with endurable pain and limited pleasure, with reasonable success and manageable failure, and with a clear conscience to tread the delicate paths of life.

O god! Guide me towards the future so that I will work for a living instead of living like a parasite on society. Let me not feel jealousy of those who work hard and progress.

O omniscient god! Enlighten those who speak in your name that neither you wrote any scripture for mankind nor did your prophets do it nor anyone authorized by you compiled the scriptures. Scriptures were written by later generations in the name of god and prophets with interpolations, deviations, additions, etc. according to the perceptions of the writers which may be different from what you taught. Enlighten mankind so that I am not forced to follow that part of the scripture, which is against my conscience but written in your name.

O god, the omnipotent and the immaculate! Let me not be under any illusion that you cannot withstand any criticism from my enemies or you are frail and fall apart before non-believers and I have to defend you with all the might to silence them.

O god, the omniscient! I respect those atheists whom I cannot answer rationally about everything that is going on in the name of the 'will of god', but I despise the behaviour of those who claim to be your devotees and do many things in your name without conscience.

O god! By donating liberally for the rituals or for a grand abode for you, let me not think that I have purchased you and you would do anything at my bidding always!

O god, the wisest! Give me the wisdom that I should do good work to go to heaven and, hiding my sin, I should not hoodwink you with some rituals, prayers, etc. to go to heaven. Also, give me the wisdom and conscience so that I do not go in search of holy rivers already overflowing with sins.

O god! Let me die a death without the burden of conscience and without burden to anyone.

DEATH

All living things including human beings are born and, at the end of their life, die in different times, fixed by providence which is beyond the cognizance of anyone. What holds the body that it is active? After death, why is the body inactive? Is there any spirit inside our body? What happens to the spirit which made the body active?

Is there anything after death or before birth? Science has delayed death, but it could not discover anything beyond death.

Human imagination and logical thinking lead to many theories about life after death. Since none can know anything beyond death and only god may do anything after death, great philosophers and social reformers brought some accountability in life. A good life would be rewarded by god after death in heaven or in the next birth.

The instinct for survival and the unpredictability of death has led to many theories and many gods embodying the social values and encouraging the followers to imbibe the social ethos.

The necessity of disposing the dead body, which may spread diseases also, leads to the framing of rules and regulations on disposing the body after death.

Criminal elements also exploited the society by promising to take the dead to heaven by doing some rituals. The gullible society was warned that, if the rituals were not done, the dead one's spirit may wander in the earth, haunting the relatives.

If anyone can show life after death with a reasonable proof, the life on earth may become strange—either anarchy if no punishment is there or peaceful and blissful if reward for good work is promised.

Since each one is born to die, why not enrich life with good thinking and wise efforts so that we can leave a better world for the future generation?

AFTER DEATH: MOVING TOWARDS HEAVEN

The spirit which activated our body has gone after death. Where does it go? Is there any life after death? Since the urge to live is innate, the fear of the unknown death is natural.

In spite of the uncertainties and unpredictable perturbations in one's life, the broad parameters that define one's life is the same. The hunger and cravings, the anger and assertions, the labour and achievements, the fight and greediness, etc. that shape the personality of a person define the broad parameters of one's life in almost all situations. God or nature has endowed all animals including human beings with an urge to survive even though death is inevitable.

Even though death is certain, just like many events in life, death is unpredictable. Death is like a black hole which attracts and assimilates anyone who wanders nearby without knowing its whereabouts.

But the law of nature is different. There is neither a perpetual donor nor a perpetual recipient. A withering tree gives enough seeds before its death, whereas a dormant seed gives birth to a living tree.

The spirit that entered the darkness of death must come out into light to play its role in a different form with different levels of maturity.

When death is certain, why not we live a reasonable life? If our spirit goes to heaven, why not let it rest in peace instead of repenting for what it has done while enlivening our body?

In a world full of chaos, an ideal life may not be possible. But if our spirit has to go to heaven, let it go in an honourable way by doing good work in its lifetime in this world without hoodwinking neither gods by shortcuts like rituals and ceremonies nor the people who trusted them.

If hell is there, why not overcome it in this life itself within the boundaries of the urge to live and the judgement of conscience and reason?

But where is heaven and hell? They are in this life itself—in the form of wife or husband, son or daughter, money, power, fame, illness, state of mind, etc. An unfaithful spouse can make the life of a person a hell; a caring son or daughter can make the life of an old man a heaven even without material comforts in life; a blunder done early in life may haunt a person till the death of the person, putting him in hell; in spite of all the comforts at one's disposal, a person may not be able to sleep because of the haunting past memories; Even though a person is having unfathomable wealth, he is living more on medicines than on food, keeping him away from heaven; playing with friends even without essential facilities may make the mind long for that heaven; an unprofessional handling of a student in the school may make the life in the school a hell; and so on.

Never underestimate your gods and goddesses – whether they are idols, stones, figures, ghost based on scriptures, god without figure. Do not befool yourself by thinking that by doing some rituals before death or by your children after death, your gods and goddesses will ignore what you have done in your life and they will be pleased only with your rituals. If you believe in heaven, try to go there in an honourable way by doing good work rather than pleasing or bribing your gods with some rituals or offerings.

Does the spirit which activates our body like an idle or ideal life after death? If the law of conservation of energy is taken as an analogy, then life can take different forms to activate a life in another body—not necessarily a human body. So heaven and hell are in this world only and there may not be any heaven or hell after death.

DEATH AND RITUALS

Just like any animal in this world, god or nature ordained man to die fighting for survival and his dead body to be used as food for scavenging animals. But man has protected himself too much that his flesh would not be available for any animal to eat. But the rotten flesh of the dead will lead to the spread of many diseases for those who are living. It has to be disposed of at the earliest, and the society has offered help in the form of mandatory rituals and ceremonies.

Do you think that the rituals and ceremonies that your descendants and family members do will help you to go to heaven?

Do you think that your god is so foolish that it will ignore your performance done throughout your life and will be pleased to allow you to reside in heaven simply because of your supplication and rituals before and after death?

The rituals after death can help to avoid diseases which may spread if the petrified body is kept for long after death. So never believe those rituals and ceremonies which will drain your money or time and which will greatly affect your future.

IMITATION OF THE LAW OF CONSERVATION OF ENERGY

As man was searching or hunting for food in the forest just like any other animal, he found that natural players like the sun, moon, wind, rain, etc. play a major role in finding food or prey. So he started worshipping these pagan gods by eulogizing or flattering them to help to find food, to provide security, etc.

As time passed, he found that the 'spirit' inside the body does everything, and if it leaves the body, the body will become rotten and fit to be thrown away for scavengers like eagles.

As man was part of a big society, he started doing many things desirable or inimical to the society. Various theories were formed according to the nature and experiences of the society to bring some accountability to the conduct of man in the society. In case he fails to get rewards or punishment in this world for his conduct, his spirit would get perpetual reward or punishment in heaven or hell.

But where does the spirit go after death? Does it go to heaven or hell or mingle with god?

Since one is paid back in the same coin in the form of a spouse, children, health, wealth, happiness, etc., the concept of heaven and hell is not tenable outside the planet Earth.

If god were the embodiment of perfection, the spirit of a '*fallible*' man cannot integrate with god in spite of his offerings, flatteries, eulogies, and other material sacrifices.

If one sees the abnormal increase of humans and the abnormal decrease of other animals in this world, one can conclude that the spirit is reborn in this world—it may be any living thing, including a human being. So, one can state the hypothesis on conservation of spirits as follows: The spirit in a body can neither be created nor destroyed, but it can transform into one form or another in this world.

'Death is like sleep, and birth is like awakening after sleep.'[20] If one were reborn after death, then it may be based on some form of accountability in life or a 'judgement'[21] on life, and not based on the capability to survive.

---

[20]   Thirukkural: An ancient book of 1,330 couplets in Tamil, a South Indian language.

[21]   Bible: On the Day of Judgement, god will resurrect all the dead persons and send them to heaven or hell according to what they have done in their life.

PERCEPTION

In life and about life, the perception of each one is different at any time. If different persons see an object, the perception about the object is different from person to person. The way a farmer sees a field is different while an agricultural scientist will see it in a different way and a businessman will see it in an altogether different way. The way an ordinary man sees the moon differs from the way an artist thinks about the moon; the way an astronomer observes the moon differs from the way a meteorologist thinks about the moon; etc.

For a parent, a toy may mean money, but for a child, it is a living companion. For an artist, a painting may be an expression of his inner feelings, but for another person, it may just look different from some other photograph. While many go for a pious journey, someone else sees a vast opportunity for doing business in the crowd. A farmer may see his agricultural plantation as a source of livelihood, a businessman may see it as a source of making a lot of money, an agricultural scientist may see the diseases and think about the pesticides needed to control it, a worker may see it as a source of earning, a child may see it as a wonderful ground to play, and so on.

When everyone fears war, there is a person who sees an opportunity to establish his authority to extended areas; another sees an opportunity to enrich oneself by selling more arms; someone else hopes to get relief from oppressive and retrograde laws of the land; etc.

Different experiences, knowledge, beliefs, and hopes create different levels of perception which may move higher or lower depending on new experiences, new knowledge, new values, new beliefs, and new hopes. These levels of perception may also move depending on the experience, persuading skills, knowledge, and perception of others. That is, there are always gaps in the perception which can be filled with further knowledge, dreams about the future, half-truths, lies, past experiences, etc, as is done by marketing strategists.

The drive or impulse for a change in life comes not only from external factors like making money, living in comfort, etc. but also from different perceptions about life and its intrinsic attributes which may be real or imaginary.

The more one sees the world, listens to other people's experiences, and has the knowledge about others' beliefs and behaviour and dares to think about them, the more one's perception in life becomes matured.

THE ART OF SPEAKING

It does not cost anything to speak a word, and it may not require too much energy to utter a word. But while speaking, keep in mind about the word that you are speaking and the people who are listening to you. A word may shape a person, and another word may kill a person.

The words of a leader may create confidence in the minds of the people while the words of an enemy may make one angry; the sweet words of a lover may be intoxicating while the carefully worded speech of a crooked person may incite a person to do bad things; the imperfect words of a child may sound like the best music while the harsh words of a master may be stinging; and a person in trouble may be consoled by a kind word while another word may make that person sleepless.

As the social or official hierarchy goes higher and higher, each word that a person utters becomes weighted more and more, and consequently, it may affect the life of many people in one way or the other or create wonderful things or bring great catastrophes. So a responsible person has to be more careful while uttering a word. 'A burn injury due to a fire may get cured, but a wound inflicted by a word may never get cured.'[22]

---

[22] Thirukkural: An ancient literature in Tamil, a South Indian language.

So learn the art of speaking, by mixing with good people in the society, and, by speaking the right word after knowing their state of mind at any time. The art of communicating one's feelings will make the family a happy family.

THE FEELING OF BEING IMPORTANT

The feeling of being important is an effect of one's ego on the mind. Ego is the creation of selfishness which is present in all animals for survival, security, and proliferation.

Each one has one's own importance in the society on specific places and times. Just like a small loose nut which stops a monumental machine, the importance of a seemingly insignificant person tremendously increases on specific occasions. During that time, one feels a sense of being an important member of the family or the society, whose contribution is essential for the well-being of the family or the society.

On any big event or special function, a recognition, that each one is treated as important and essential, makes a lot of difference in making the function a success and in doing any future work without much problem. A casual talk, a sense of recognition through gesture, an appreciation of a past event done by a person, recollecting childhood pranks, etc. will surely enhance one's self-esteem while talking with friends and relatives and accept through one's heart that it is the personal function of everyone.

A neglected person may be able to create chaos in an organised function or in normal work on some specific time or place. A neglected Eris[23] was able to create a commotion in a crowd that eventually led to the devastating Trojan War. A person neglected to loneliness may explode with the grievances in the family or the society.

The feeling of being important is a natural mindset, but claiming to be the most important person and claiming to the privileges associated with it may cause more problems for the family and the society on some occasions.

---

[23] Eris, a Greek goddess of discord was not invited deliberately for the nuptials of Peleus, a king, and Thetis, a nymph. Eris dropped a golden apple for the fairest woman in the crowd which led to a chain of events including the Trojan War. The Trojan war was between the Greeks and the City of Troy and it lasted for 10 years.

SUCCESS AND FAILURE

Everyone's life is destined in such a way that neither success nor failure is perpetual even if the person is very good or very bad. It is also true for a society or a country, but it may take more time for a country compared to individuals.

Success is a psychological booster, but successive successes are intoxicating and sedative, whereas successive failures are demoralizing and humiliating.

Also, success for one person may be a failure for someone else. One learns from both success and failure, and this learning really shapes the thinking and behaviour. Due to successive successes, one may become arrogant since he may feel invincible, and in the process, he may lose his friends and family. Successive failures may make a person docile, and he may lose faith in his abilities.

For success in any field, knowledge, planning, and perseverance help. But luck, in the form of an unknown providential intervention in time, also helps. Had not Napoleon Bonaparte[24] suffered severe stomach ache, the Battle of Waterloo may have been different. At least, one

---

[24] Napoleon Bonaparte, an emperor of France who used to start war early, started war at Waterloo late due to severe stomach ache. That helped the forces of British General Arthur Wellesley and the forces of Prussian Field Marshal Gebhard Leberecht von Blücher to come closer.

may hope, he might have been more cautious in Waterloo while committing his elite troops to charge an enemy in high ground if he were there in the battlefield instead of his deputy.

Proper education, whether formal or informal, good manners, and a good environment in the house and in the society where one lives are essential for a successful life. 'Success by any means' or 'success anyhow' may lead to immorality, vice, or corruption. Success is just a means to achieve our goal, and success is not a goal in itself.

Since success and failure are part of life, gloating over success or feeling dejected over failure may not lead to a successful life. The pleasure of success is not everlasting, and the pain of failure drains out in the course of time. A success may lead to a series of failure in life and vice versa.

Some failures are turning points in history. A failure may lead to a more cautious and more planned approach in life.

If god or nature has created the living and nonliving things on earth, then it has to keep everything in balance by giving an opportunity to win or lose. So a perpetual victory for anyone is against the law of god or nature. A successful person does not get everything in life nor a failed person loses everything in life.

Of course, success in one's endeavour does not guarantee a comfortable life[25].

---

[25] Charles Goodyear, an American inventor invented the process of vulcanisation of rubber and patented it. This has revolutionized the transportation industry by producing quality tyres. But, he died a pauper.

TIME AS A PART OF EACH GOAL

Time is a part of each goal or achievement. It is an important factor in enhancing or diminishing the effect of achievement, just like the hot news of a news paper or old news paper.

If shown after adulthood, the love and affection which ought to have been shown to a child may be embarrassing.

Offering a glass of water to a thirsty person is far more valuable than offering litres of water later. Offering a glass of water to a person choked with food has more impact than taking that person to a hospital later.

A few minutes of consoling a person at a moment of defeat has a far more positive effect than hours of counselling later.

A few minutes of first aid to an accident victim in time far outweighs hours of surgery done later in saving a life.

It is too late to realize, if an old man feels that he should have looked after his father when he was old and feeble.

When one achieves a goal and stops in its glory, someone else overtakes that achievement in the course of time.

A few seconds of time may differentiate a winner from a loser in a running race.

A person in his twenties and another in his sixties may get the same degree from an university at the same time but their significances are quite different because of the time lag.

FAILURE AND SUPPORT

At any time in an ideal situation, the chance for success is hardly 1 per cent, whereas it is more than 99 per cent for failure. Only one can win a race among the competitors after years of training; only one can become the prime minister of a country after spending so much time and money to convince the people; only one can be made the head of an institution among the hundreds of applicants; only one team can win in a tournament of football in a country; and so on. Proper training, investment, perseverance, etc. are paid back in the form of success, fame, a chance to live a comfortable life, and above all, a sense of self-satisfaction. But the cost of failure is too high to bear for many people.

The world being vast with opportunities to accommodate more people, many people may succeed in life at the same time. Many persons may get employment to do a single work as in assembling a big machine; many may find a single, but cheap, mode of transport to go to work; many pupils may pass the examination and go to the next level; many persons may become doctors and go to work in different cities and towns; and so on. Everyone gets a chance to live a decent life, but there is always a craving for something more to do or achieve.

Some people plan and invest everything they have—money, time, labour, etc.—and work for success. When they fail, they find the world humiliating and not worth living. Friends and acquaintances mock at the idea. Financiers demand money immediately, fearing the nonrefund of money, and a failed person finds nowhere to go for support and sustenance. If such a failed person gets moral or material support from a friend or a relative or a well-wisher, he can rise again and stand on his own leg in the same, or in a different, endeavour. But who will bet on a losing horse? There may be someone who believes in the ability and the talent of a person even after failure hits hard. Such a person is surely a lucky one!

MISTAKE

More work leads to more mistakes.
Less work leads to less mistakes.
No work leads to no mistake.

So an active life means more mistakes or, in other words, more experiences. Even careful planning leads to failure sometimes. Even a hundred successful launches of rockets do not guarantee the successful launch of the next one. A well-trained pilot may fumble in a foggy weather. A smart and experienced driver may meet with an accident. Even a careful weeding out of weeds will leave some weeds unharmed in a garden. Even careful nurturing of saplings may not help it to survive because of some known or unknown mistakes.

To err is human, but to go on erring is criminal. Let us learn from mistakes to avoid future mistakes and to correct ourselves. For success in life, planning and an error-free execution of the plan are essential. The human effort to remove mistakes and renovate things has lead to great success, both for survival and progress.

A hundred per cent perfection in all work is neither possible nor desirable. Had god created the world perfectly, then earth might have been smooth and polished without the hills, valleys, and rivers; all men and women might have looked alike with the same character without any heroes and adventurers; there might be only one pleasant season without the hot summer or shivering winter; there may be only day without any night; and so on.

When there is a shortage of time to think or to do, as in the case of an emergency or while doing any work in a hurry, the chances for doing mistakes are more. Lack of knowledge or training may also cause more mistakes. More than anything else, lack of enough sleep causes a lot of mistakes in one's work including incomplete learning in a school, careless mistakes in an examination, traffic accidents, etc. Strangely enough, those with less knowledge and wisdom do less mistakes, but those who presume that they have more knowledge and wisdom commit more blunders.

When a heavy tool slips and falls on the ground, it is a mistake, but when it falls on someone's head, one commits a blunder. So try to avoid mistakes even though to err is human.

MISTAKE AND OPPORTUNITY

If each mistake deserves an equally severe punishment, there may be none left out in this world without being maimed or killed. Even after so much generous pardon and the benefit of the doubt given to each and everyone doing mistakes, no one has become a perfect person after learning from past mistakes.

One's mistake is another's opportunity. A lion which raises its head a few seconds earlier by mistake gives an opportunity for the deer to survive. A mistake of a doctor to diagnose an ailment may be an opportunity for another doctor to establish one's name in the society. The mistake of a lawyer not to quote some past judgements might have given an opportunity to the other side to win. The mistake of a scientist not to publish his research findings in time might have given an opportunity to some other scientists to establish their names.

A careless mistake of one student may give an opportunity to another student to come first in an examination. A second's thought to pull the trigger by a policeman may give an opportunity for the robber to escape. The over-confidence of a politician and his inaction may give an opportunity to his opponent to contact the electorate in person and win.

Had not Hitler invaded Soviet Union[26] or had not Japan attacked Pearl Harbour,[27] the course of World War II might have been different.

A small mistake may create a major impact, just like a small loose screw may stop a giant machine.

At the same time, one may be oblivious to a big mistake which, in the course of time, may lead to a major change in life.

---

[26]   Hitler invaded Soviet Union soon after defeating the British and French armies and the withdrawal of British forces from Dunkirk leaving their tanks, artillery, and heavy weapons in France. He thought that the British can be won easily with the help of the air force and submarines, called U-boats. It gave breathing space for Britain.

[27]   Even though the United States proclaimed neutrality initially, it was helping Britain militarily through the Lend-Lease programme. After the Japanese attacked Pearl Harbor, a naval facility of the US in the Pacific, the United States entered the war on the side of Allied Powers which dramatically changed the course of the war.

MISTAKE AND PUNISHMENT

If the mistakes are common, then appropriate punishments should be rare. Also, if a person does a mistake and repents later, that person should be given an opportunity to reform himself without getting undue advantage accrued due to his past mistakes. Punishment should be limited if the confessions come from the core of one's heart. Some people may take this as undue advantage and indulge in doing mistakes, thinking that they would get the benefit of the doubt and escape punishment.

When a person does not learn from past mistakes and does not try to avoid mistakes in future or correct the wrongdoings, that person becomes bold in doing mistakes, with confidence in mind in escaping from punishment. Thus, criminals are shaped based on the response they got from their families and the society. If the family and the society respond positively and try to correct the person in time, the society will flourish as a civil society.

Each mistake or blunder leaves some invisible impressions on the minds of others, and it may leave some implicit or explicit evidence. It is for the society to decide whether to follow the trail of evidence or not.

Strangely enough, for a person with a conscience, punishment is not needed, but for a criminal, only punishment is useless.

Since no one wants to live a life of a criminal, it is the care given by the family and the society and the moral values cherished by the individual and the society that determine whether anyone wants to do mistakes continuously.

Since no one likes to live with a criminal, both counselling and partial segregation are necessary to reform a criminal. Even then, as long as punishment is not a psychological deterrent from doing mistakes, many selfish members in the society may create anarchy.

If the progeny of Adam—that is, the progeny of god's own creation—had to be punished with the Deluge, is it possible for the progeny of Noah,[28] who are, after all, a man's creation, to escape punishment? If one deserves punishment, is death the only punishment? Besides the dreaded corporeal punishments, there are punishments inflicting psychological pain through harsh words, denying sensual pleasures like hearing music, seeing a favourite film, etc.

Of course, there is no guarantee for a reward in life for each good work, nor is there some sort of punishment for each wrongdoing.

---

[28] Old Testament: Noah was a good man, and he was saved by god from heavy rain lasting for forty days with a help of a great ship known as Noah's ark. Except Noah and his wife, the rest of mankind in the world died in the Deluge as punishment for their sins.

FORGIVENESS

As the saying goes, 'To err is human but to forgive is divine.' To forgive those who realize their mistakes is divine. But to forgive those who do mistakes deliberately to harm others is callous. Do those who go on doing mistakes deserve forgiveness?

No one is perfect. Naturally, mistakes are common in behaviour, in speech, in doing things, in perceiving, in thinking, etc.

If every mistake deserves punishment, there may be none left without being punished, humiliated, fined, maimed, killed, etc. A good society gives an opportunity to live a reformed life if a criminal repents for what he did.

Who really feels sorry for the mistake done? Who really deserves forgiveness? Is it to those who wail and shout, proclaiming that they have really realized their mistakes? Is it to those who really feel for their mistakes and change their behaviour and outlook? Of course, each one has one's own judgement in forgiving others.

There are occasions when we do make mistakes, sometimes against our own judgement and sometimes against the social values cherished by the society. Are we honest till we are caught for the mistakes? Can we forgive ourselves by justifying what we did, or will our conscience haunt us forever? Will the society forgive us if we tell the truth about the wrongs done, or will it throw stones[29] at us? Are our misdeeds and ill-thoughts pardonable at the altar of our conscience or social etiquette?

When the system is corrupt or the social institutions are corrupt and one is forced to do wrong things, who will forgive those who are trapped in the corrupt system?

---

[29] Bible: Killing by throwing stones at the sinner was a custom in a society. When a sinner was about to be stoned to death, Jesus Christ told the crowd that the one who did not commit any sin should come forward to throw the first stone. Since the crowd had been enlightened and each one had a conscience, none came forward, and the person accused of sin was pardoned.

ENEMY AND PROTECTION

A person may have a few friends, but nature has given a lot of enemies besides the enemies that one creates for oneself. The enemy may be as big as an elephant or as small as a mosquito or a virus.

Strangely enough, the wind that helps to move faster will start opposing the movement from the moment the speed increases more than the speed of the wind. So if there is no enemy, then the enemy is created automatically. If there is no physical enemy, man creates his own enemy in the mind with devastating consequences.

With the probability of big or small enemies all round being more, none is provided 100 per cent protection. Of course, the level of protection may vary according to the physical environment or mental state of each and every person. A fortified fortress may protect a person for a long time, but it may not be possible to protect oneself from a resourceful enemy forever.

When the enemies form a critical network against a good person, the loss to the society, in terms of physical and psychological contributions, is immense. Such evil persons in the society—even though victorious—become morally bankrupt, but the society cannot free itself from their shackles for a long time.

Suspicion, misunderstanding, fear, vanity and selfishness create more enemies than one can face.

Exposing what others want to hide, forcing to do when one is reluctant to do, doing what others cannot tolerate, and preaching what others fear to understand due to selfishness are the main causes for making enemies. Socrates created more enemies by exposing the ignorance of the influential sophists in the society, and ultimately, he was poisoned to death[30].

As the number of enemies increases, the protective physical and psychological coatings that one is having are prickled, creating uneasiness in life and sometimes creating devastating consequences.

---

[30] Socrates, an ancient Greek Philosopher used dialogue-questioning just like an ignorant and eliciting answers from others, and ultimately establishing his views or exposing his opponents. In this way, he exposed the powerful and the rich of their hoary believes, vanity, boastfulness etc. They ganged against Socrates and charged him for impiety and for spoiling the youths of Athens, a city state and condemned him to death.

THE JOY OF DAYDREAMING

The gap between reality and expectation is so large that it is difficult to achieve the dream in most of the cases. But a person's ingenuity in fulfilling the expectations is found in the joy of daydreaming—that is, the joy of achieving one's goal without even having a glimpse of the hurdles and dangers associated with the goal in reality.

Who would not like to win a war without any casualty or win a tournament against a local champion without proper preparation, or come first in an examination without studying hard, or become the cynosure of all eyes in a party, or challenge and subdue a local thug who creates nuisance in the locality, or scale new heights in an adventure, or be a hero or heroine before the opposite sex?

If there were no daydreaming, there would be no fascinating fairy tales or interesting stories and novels or good films. A person identifies himself with the main character in the story and feels sad when the main character is in trouble or exuberant when the hero or heroine wins and morally supports when the main character toils against insurmountable problems.

But to achieve the goal in reality, there is no alternative to hard and wise work. Of course, a supportive family, good books, good friends, proper planning, etc. may help in achieving one's dreams.

To get a treasure which was saved by someone else or win a raffle that is the contribution of thousands of similar people, gambling one's way to riches, etc. may be liked by all. But the treasure may be the outcome of the hard work of many people for many years. If everyone likes the easy way of achieving everything in life through daydreaming, who will generate wealth by hard work? Is it possible to do it through share-market?

One prefer to hear what one likes. So, politicians convert our dreams into their votes through promises of our liking. Who would like a person who says that your dream is unrealistic?

GOOD AND BAD

Good and bad things in life are defined by the society and the family for the welfare of the members of the society.

Good rules should be followed, and good behaviour is to be appreciated. The ultimate reward for doing good things in life is that the gateway to heaven would open after death and god would bestow abundance of good things in life on those who are good.

On the other hand, for doing bad and sinful things in life, there is the threat of going to hell after death.

What is good or bad differs from society to society, and within the same society, it changes with time. Killing a man in the society is bad, but killing an enemy—a euphemism for an outsider—is appreciated as bravery. Dying in a war with the enemy may help one to go to heaven in a society, whereas in another society, war and killings may lead to perpetual birth with a lot of indignities to suffer in future. Stories of killing a giant—a euphemism for a man in a different society—and looting his property is always heard with admiration in all societies. People are conditioned to do what is good and not to do bad things because of the reward in heaven and the punishment in hell.

What is good or bad? There is no strict demarcation in the 'state of nature'[31], but when the humans started living in different societies, moral values associated with the well being of each society define the good and the bad for that society, some of them were more humane and a few of them were more dogmatic. So, good and bad always depends on the context, the situation, the time, and above all, the society. Beating a thief and beating a good person may not be the same unless the law treats both of them equal.

Since change is the order of the world, as time passes, what are perceived as good and bad dogmas really choke the society until there is a saviour who dares to lead them towards the light.

---

[31] John Locke, a British Philosopher talks about a situation when men in '…a state of perfect freedom to order their actions, and dispose of their possessions and persons, as they think fit, within the bounds of the law of nature, without asking leave, or depending upon the will of any other man….' That is, he talks about the natural environment in which primitive man, who was born selfish and struggled for survival alone before the formation of cooperative living or society, lived.

HONESTY

Is there anyone who does not want to be honest? Of course, none. But selfishness, greediness, and vanity make almost everyone to succumb to the pressure of dishonesty. Different societies condoned dishonesty many times when it suited them.

Honesty is lonely and inflexible, and hence, it is always a prey to all types of vices. The honest King Harishchandra[32], who used to keep his word, was hounded by a beggar called Vishwamitra and humiliated. A few criminals and unscrupulous people in the society utilized such stories to suppress the honest society and exploited them. Strangely enough, in a direct fight between an honest person and a vicious person, many vicious forces gang against the honest person to ensure the victory of the wicked person.

In a society, if the majority is honest, the society progresses. But when the majority is dishonest or when a few dishonest people can suppress the majority psychologically or through violence, the society becomes so corrupt that people start justifying anything for selfish

---

[32] An ancient Sanskrit story in India: Vishwamitra begged King Harishchandra to donate his kingdom, and after getting the kingdom, he put Harishchandra under many difficulties and humiliation. The king had to sell himself and his wife to keep his word and suffered till the end.

reasons, and the society loses all moral values. A family which forbids criticism or a society which is intolerant to criticism, whatever the justification be, moves away from honest living.

If one has an opportunity to act dishonestly and none is likely to catch that person, will that person act honestly? If one is not honest, none can prevent him from becoming dishonest whenever the opportunity arises. So, honesty depends on the values cherished by a person and his trust in the society as its member. So corruption starts in the minds of man and his belief in circumventing the society. Once one succumbs to corruption, the risk of exposure of corruption is so great that one is trapped further in a series of corrupt practices and criminal activities.

One can be honest only if one believes in working for a living and living within one's means. Greediness and delaying work beyond limit breeds corruption.

In life, strangely enough, honest people are forced to do wrong things due to circumstances, particularly by corrupt systems or institutions of the society. Also, by the time dishonest people repent for their past and change their minds, it is too late in their lives. Strangely enough, in a fight between virtue and vice, the vice wins most of the time, most probably to enjoy the fruits of its misdeeds immediately and experience the pangs of success later. Sane voices are rarely heard in time.

A corrupt person may change and, out of remorse, do honest work in a later life, but it is very difficult for an honest person to do the right thing in a corrupt system. A corrupt system in a society will make an honest person suffer for ever as Harishchandra had to endure, and the honest person has to adjust himself into the corrupt system against one's own conscience. The moral superiority of the society can be judged by the system of governing the society and its successful management. A good system of governance or management includes subsystems for self-monitoring and prompt correction when something goes wrong.

A person who does not believe in work for a living and who does not save a little for future uncertainties can hardly live honestly.

ONE IN A MILLION

Among the millions of persons in the society, I love my mother who cares for me. I appreciate the man who dared to challenge a criminal, risking his own life. I like the Good Samaritan[33] who helped a man who met with an accident. I like the doctor who tried her level best to save a life. I appreciate the boy who removed a stone lying on the road and hindering traffic. I like that person who dared to explore the unknown world. I appreciate the person who toiled day and night to complete the work. I appreciate the girl who answered all the questions of the teacher. I like the bureaucrat who did the work honestly, circumventing the red tape.

Among the millions of persons in the society, I like the author who gave a real picture of the society. I appreciate the leader who differed with the masses and tried to lead them in the right direction. I revere the man who could have humiliated his opponent but who forgave his enemy and treated him with honour. I revere the teacher who taught me more than what he ought to teach. I love the person who helped me while I was in trouble; and my regards go to the old man who gave practical advice to

---

[33] Bible: A traveller was wounded by thieves. Many passers-by, including pious persons, went without helping him. A Good Samaritan cleaned his wounds and provided necessary help.

follow in life. I admire the person who remained honest even though he got ample opportunity to swindle money without being caught. I appreciate the police officer who has collected the evidence and regenerated the events leading to the crime. I respect my teacher who took pains to correct me when I did wrong in the company of bad friends. I like the person who spoke a few kind words while I was in trouble.

But why am I not one among them? Of course, it is because of my selfishness.

ONE AMONG THE CROWD

I could have helped the man who was bleeding due to an accident, but I did not help since I was one of the spectators who did not have any relationship with him. I could have done more for my students, but I did not do so since I would not gain anything for the extra work. As a public servant, I could have answered politely to those who asked for details, but I did not do so since there was none to question me.

I could have taught the student who failed in the examination separately, but I did not do that since I was not going to gain anything from that. As a witness, I could have told the truth before the judge about what the criminal had done to the good person, but I did not do so since the threat of the criminal was haunting me. I could have desisted from taking a bribe from anyone, but I did not do so since the lure of comfort and pleasure was tempting me, and also, who could prove that I took the bribe? As a lawyer, I could have advised my client not to file a court case, but I did not do so since I was earning more by the court case. I could have helped the public by advising my juniors to do their work in time, but I did not do so since I was afraid of my juniors' murmurs and loud protests.

As a doctor, I could have prescribed only the required medicines based on the symptoms to my patient, but I also suggested scanning and blood tests so that I could get a commission from the clinical laboratory. I could have handed over the costly camera that I found in the park to the police, but I did not do so since none knew that I took it. I could have advised the workers not to go on strike, but I did not do so since I wanted to harass the company manager who questioned me for coming late to office regularly.

Even though I could have done things with professional ethics or common sense, I failed to do so because of selfishness or fear, and hence, I was standing just like any other person in the crowd.

SELFISHNESS VERSUS SERVICE

Even though man is the last animal in the series of evolution, man is born selfish just like any other animal. So, there is hardly anyone whose only motive is doing any service except a few who are really concerned about the course followed by the family or the society.

A bee is not doing any service to a tree by cross-pollinating, but it is only interested in gathering honey for itself. The service to a tree is done by cross-pollinating unintentionally in spite of the selfishness of the bee.

Selfishness is not perfectly moulded and sealed. Money preserved by a miser may find its way to others through the spouse, children, friends, or through some rituals. Selectively watering plants in the garden may also find its way to weeds in the garden.

It is the enlightened selfishness, where people are ready to sacrifice some of their selfishness for the sake of a group of people, that helped the formation of society and its institutions were sustained. For the protection of the society, people were even ready to fight with enemies and die.

So when anyone does work, the value of the product increases depending on the selfish value attached to the work. Enlightened selfishness attaches a less selfish value while greedy people attach more profit even if the product is for a social welfare scheme. A small farmer may attach a small value for his produce, whereas a businessman may attach more value and sell for more profit.

ACHIEVEMENT

Achievement is, indeed, wonderful in life. There is nothing in life which is free. Someone or the other should pay or work for that.

When everyone is sleeping, achievers toil even in night; when everyone is talking, they think; when everyone is enjoying during a festival, they wait for a customer; when everyone is playing safely, they take the risk; when everyone is fearing, they dare and challenge; when everyone searches for a path, they move ahead of others, creating a path; when everyone thinks of the present, they think of the future based on the experience of the past or with a hope for the future; when everyone dreams of Utopia[34], they sail for it; when everyone follows the mob, they leave a different trail; etc.

The knowledge that the human beings have attained and the comfort that they are enjoying are because of the cumulative achievements made by different achievers in different fields like science, arts, commerce, politics, etc., sacrificing many things dear to them.

No doubt, the risks involved are more. Sometimes, any failure may cost their life. But what is really painful would be when people make them the laughing stock when they fail.

---

[34] A book by Thomas More: Utopia is an imaginary island where everything is perfect and people are reasonable.

THE COST OF ACHIEVEMENT

The achievement in life comes with resource, plan, effort, and time playing major roles. But what is the cost of achievement?

Excellence is achieved in any field by sacrificing something dear. The cost of achievement is to be paid in terms of time, physical or mental labour, loneliness, separation from family, moving away from a safe and secure environment, etc.

A successful police officer may not find time to look after his children; a successful lady officer may not find time to feed her baby in time; a good administrator may not be able to sleep due to the worries about future plans; a student scoring very high marks may have no time to play his favourite game with his friends; a judge might have lost the joy of mixing with the crowd in a function; an adventurer might have left his family alone for a long time; a successful businessman might have no time to celebrate festivals; an industrialist may find no time to see a good cinema; a successful politician may not find time even to stay with his family for a few days; a scientist may not find time to guide his own children; etc.

A sportsperson wins a game after sacrificing his time and money on training in a game or sports. A mountaineer sacrifices his comfort to climb a cliff. A reformer sacrifices his time, energy, money, and sometimes, life for changing a society. A mother sacrifices her sleep and comfort to bring up her child. A scientist sacrifices his time and energy to pursue an unknown hypothesis. A doctor leaves the pleasant company of her family to attend to an ailing patient.

For an achiever, the fruits of achievement—fame, name, wealth, and the feeling of greatness—may be available later in life, but they do not come without the associated cost in terms of sacrificing comfort, sleep, money, the company of the friends and family, etc.

The risk of failure in achieving things is more which deters everyone to dare to achieve. Only talent and perseverance together with time and resource can help to achieve.

One can dream of achieving something in life without losing anything, but not in real life.

FRIEND

If birds of the same feather flock together, then the people of the same outlook and inclination befriend each other.

A person can be judged by the friends that one is having. When a person comes to a new locality, he slowly takes his place in the new environment and forms his own circle of friends in which people of his mentality are abundant.

A pent-up feeling may implode one's mind and destroy the peace of mind besides harming members in the society who are nearby. Others may exploit the feelings and the weaknesses arising out of it, but only a friend will give right ideas and help to manage the situation in a right way.

A person can influence the thinking and behaviour of his or her friend. A person who does not correct the wrong behaviour of his friend or exploits the weakness of his friend or does not show the right way to his friend cannot be a true friend. Since a slight incitement or encouragement may make a person to do wrong things easily, leading to a lot of embarrassment, a person in the company of a bad friend may find life difficult and humiliating later.

Trust your friends and be trustworthy for your friends. That is the only way to preserve your friendship. A betrayed trust costs more than the damage that an enemy could inflict, both physically and mentally. A friend who encourages wrongdoings or deserts when in trouble or leaks out confidential matters is far more dangerous than a few honest enemies. An honest enemy may have minimum norm or etiquette while an unfaithful friend may know the strength and weakness and so can cause more damage than an enemy.

A person who encourages when one's friend attempts to do something in life or soothes the feelings when a friend fails to win in an attempt or corrects the wrong path chosen by one's friend can be called a true friend.

A person has to divulge his mind or tell the problem so that the friends can help. This may sometimes create problems since a friend of today may turn out to be a foe of tomorrow. But an observer from outside may be able to see things differently and suggest better ways to tackle problems.

Remember that books and pet animals are best companions with whom one can pass the time without any fear of exploitation. But books and pet animals are not substitutes for a friend since humans are social animals. Friends are interdependent psychologically and like the company of each other.

Instant friends are neither possible nor desirable. Good people help the helpless not because of their friendship but because of their clear conscience and noble thinking. But as in fairy tales, will they come in time while one is in trouble?

CONSTRUCTION AND DESTRUCTION

Construction and destruction are part of life just like birth and death. That is, there is nothing which remains perpetually as it is. The construction and destruction may be physical or psychological.

Sometimes, individuals build wonderful things and wonderful machines or create wonderful ideas for themselves, for their families, or for the society. In the course of time, all those wonderful things are altered, modified, or even destroyed.

Sometimes, individuals, families and societies create their own values, ideas, ideals, and also idols and rituals to reinforce them. Some other individual, family or society destroys everything and imposes their own ideals as superior. After a few generations, there is a revolt destroying the foundation on which the new ideals stand. One society builds their gods and associate different values with them. After a few generations, those gods are replaced with new ones with new characteristics. Sometimes, there are revolts within the society, destroying what was shaped by the society for centuries. The Knowledge of evolution of different religions and their gods may help to understand this.

Nature also does its duty in construction and destruction. It may be a drop of water for a plant through rain, a storm destroying a tree, a volcano destroying a habitat, an earthquake destroying a town, etc.

Societies go to war, destroying or looting the valuables of the defeated and constructing a dreamland using the looted materials.

One thing that shapes man and woman more than anything else is the construction and destruction going on in the minds of individuals. Can they construct their future with a plan, effort, resources, and services and without envy, malice, ill will, etc.? Can they play a fair game for a win?

TRUST VERSUS BETRAYAL

One's mind is invisible to others. The uncertainties of events in life and the unfathomable mind have given rise to suspicion in the mind on many things in life.

There are exigencies in life when people suspect others but, even then, ask for help, reposing faith in the Almighty or humane values, as in the case of an accident. There are occasions when people trust but they are betrayed.

It is good to be trusted, and be worthy of the trust. Without trust, none can live in the society, nor can anyone give to, or take from, anyone.

Strangely enough, the history of mankind is abundant with stories of trusted people betraying and suspected people turning out to be trustworthy. Necessities and selfishness make a trusted friend of the day into a betrayer during the night, and a loyal soldier betrays his own country.

In a society where there is lack of mutual trust, it is very difficult to live. There will be suspicion and perpetual fear always, and hence, the progress towards prosperity and happiness will be limited.

If any child's trust on his parents, friends, teachers, and the members of the society is betrayed, it may lead to major abnormalities in the mind of the child which, in turn, may lead to abnormal behaviour later in life.

Trust has to be earned by words, deeds, and behaviour. Say what you will do and do not be diplomatic in real life. That is, do not play with words or do not act in real life.

Trust and betrayal go together—if there is no trust, the chances of betrayal is less, but without trust, life is hardly worth living.

PAST, PRESENT, AND FUTURE

No past lies without experience,
No present lies without belief,
No future lies without hope.

The experiences and the perception of the past and the knowledge of the present shape the *belief* of the present and the *hope or dreams* for the future.

A person with bitter experiences and limited resources is more cautious in his approach than a person who is successful. A successful person dares to do and tries to take risks with more confidence in success.

Of course, each failure is endowed with a gift of enlightenment for a person with perseverance. Of course, a person who persists with his efforts for success in a line of work may not succeed in that work, but that person may discover some other way for success in some other field. Success has multiple routes towards it, and it is multifaceted.

PAST AS A BASE FOR FUTURE

The past is a base full of knowledge and experience. Together with the effort of the present, the future of each person unfolds.

It is the wisdom gained from past knowledge and experience that one's attitude is formed, and together with the resource of the present, the dream of each person's future will be unfolded.

The past has tremendous influence on the future. A small bite from a dog may make a person always fearful of dogs, and a small piece of advice when in trouble may persist in the mind for a long time.

A person who did not face any bitter experience in the past may venture into the future more boldly.

But accepting the present without the past may cause many lacunae in future.

But how does one predict the nature of the future outcomes before venturing into it? Acquire necessary knowledge and develop skill before dreaming 'I can win'. Never leave your success to chance. Of course, there are ambiguities in life which, when ventured into, may change depending on the time, place, people, effort, and perception. Without knowing where the golden apples were, it was purely a chance for Hercules[35] to meet the right person who could bring them. Had he lost hope before meeting Atlas, all his efforts might have become mere waste.

[35] Greek Mythology: Hercules (actual Greek name is Heracles) was ordered to bring the golden apples of the Hesperides. After wandering without knowing where they were, he met Atlas, the father of the Hesperides, who agreed to bring the golden apples.

PAST AS A YOKE IN FUTURE

When the memories of the past are bitter and thoughts frequently revolve around those memories, the memories of the past will become like a yoke inhibiting the progress towards the future.

The ancients devised many techniques to make the broken hearts functional. Pardon, ablution of sin in a river, pilgrimage to a distant holy place, penance, singing songs loudly and rituals were some of them.

When the memory of the past gives sleepless nights, and if the past mistake cannot be rectified, then it is meaningless to venture into the future with the yoke of the past. Forget the past, resolve not to commit such blunder in the future, and conduct yourself with a clear conscience in future. Before that, if possible, accept the truth before those whose lives were shattered because of your conduct and behaviour and, if possible, help them reconstruct their lives. But that is a tough task.

Kindling the past may overshadow the future. Forgetting the past means disowning the present. It is really a dilemma.

MIND

The life of a person is determined by

i)   the place in which one is living.
ii) the society and the environment in which one lives.
iii) the beliefs and hopes that shape a person.

Among these, it is the beliefs and hopes that dominate in deciding the course of life in an adult. It is the mind which tells how to behave with a friend or with a foe; how to treat a stranger—as a good or bad person; how to behave with a neighbour—as an indifferent person or as a friend; etc.

The mind, at any time, is the product, primarily, of the input given to the brain through the senses—eyes, ears, nose, mouth and the body. The input may be as old as a story from a friend in childhood or as recent as a news in an electronic medium or the way the father or mother treated the person while he or she was an infant.

Since the inputs are dynamic, in addition to the existing volume of raw and processed data, various combinations and recombinations occur, resulting in a fluid mind and associated thinking. One can be convinced easily with additional input to change the way of thinking.

The input from reliable sources like parents, friends, reputed persons, etc. has far more importance in shaping the mind than those from other sources.

In general, the mind will have thoughts based on the dominating input. Since the eyes and ears input voluminous data into the brain compared to other senses, the impact on the thought process due to what we see and hear is enormous.

The state of the conscious mind at any time is like a dynamic fluid always moving like a curve, with singularities causing discontinuity or abnormal changes in the thought process. The thought process in the mind is mostly broken by sensual feelings like hunger, touch, sight, etc. If the intensity of the thought is more, the sensuous stimulus should be more to break the course of thought, just like a loud noise.

A broken thought in the mind changes its direction or subject of thought or both.

A normal state of mind indicates a normal thought and associated behaviour and activities.

An excited state of mind is an energized state which has a potential to do more physical and mental activities, both positive and negative.

A frigid state of mind is a condition in which one resists to think beyond a closed boundary of thought, and hence, the physical and mental activities are minimal.

Sensual inputs like food, assuring words, etc. or the promise of sensual gratification can change the state of mind to an excited state with a lot of potential to do things both physically and mentally.

An excited state of mind with sufficient knowledge and capabilities can do wonders in this world.

CONSCIENCE

A conscience is a judgement about oneself based on one's beliefs and values. Because of the conditioning in the society, social values, and ethics normally supersede individual values.

Man being the last animal in the series of evolution, selfishness and hence the ego are innate. To suppress the pricking conscience, war was justified in the name of gods. Deliberate critical delay or tampering an instrument was labelled as unknown cause, just to cause trouble or to take revenge on someone. Conscience is the only witness which was passive when the values imbibed by oneself or the society were trampled with impunity. So a conscience-stricken person corrects himself even if there is none to catch him.

Due to conscience, many social reformers and political thinkers rose against established social evils which were followed for centuries. Most of them had made an impact in the society, if not immediately, in the course of time.

Since the values of a society differ from place to place and the values of a person differ from person to person because of different experiences and perceptions about life, the impact of conscience differs from person to person.

Conscience is a witness against oneself when one has done something wrong, or it is a one-man army against the whole society when one feels what is done by the society is not right.

It is the conscience which has turned criminals into trustees of welfare measures. If there is a person of conscience, there is also a person of easy virtue who easily washes the sin through some rituals and ceremonies for perpetual vicious exploitation or selfishness.

If the conscience is a touchstone for doing any deed or for speaking any word, then there would not be any conflict in this world.

The conscience is dwarfed by selfishness many times, but selfishness is also dwarfed by the conscience sometimes.

Selfishness can blunt the conscience, and the conscience manifests when selfish needs are fulfilled.

PEACE OF MIND

Peace of mind is a normal state of mind where conscience, reason, personal values and social etiquette are balanced.

The past and the future are a continuum through the present, with the present as the outcome of the past and the future which is based on the perceptions of the past, the realities of the present, and dreams about the future.

Ensure that the past does not haunt you, because of some omissions and commissions magnified beyond proportion, so as to spoil the future. A clear conscience is the best source of peace of mind. Be empathetic while dealing with others, for any one can slip or falter at any moment.

Prefer to have the company of good friends or honest people who dare to say on your face that you are wrong when you are wrong.

It is better to have the company of books or pursue some hobbies rather than enjoying in the company of bad friends. The enjoyment may become a nightmare.

Lack of time is a source of tension. While doing any work, take a reasonable time for completion, or associate more resources and services for a timely completion.

Next to time pressure, lack of sleep causes more tension. Lack of sleep causes more mistakes, and so, it takes more time to complete any work properly, including mental work. Have enough sleep. An adult needs approximately eight to ten hours of sleep daily for maintaining the body and mind.

When tension and worries haunt your mind, check whether you can find a solution within your means and with the resources at your disposal. If not, it is of no use to worry about what you cannot do. In that case, be prepared to leave it to god or time and flow with the wind without bothering about the course, and be prepared to bear the outcome. Of course, there is no alternative. Pray, for time is the best healer and soothes the mind.

Prefer to tell your worries to your trustworthy friends. They may show some innovative ways.

Sing loudly and, if possible, chit-chat with your friends on simple matters. That may take off your worries and looping thoughts from the mind for some time. Initiate talk with people, preferably with family members or friends, on noncontroversial topics.

Avoid being static. Try to move to a nearby place or plan a tour. That may take off some worries. Idleness bloats tension beyond proportions. If the causes of tension can be changed, delve into it to face the challenge since none can escape from tension altogether.

When under tension, prefer to do simple physical work like gardening which does not need concentration of the mind.

Many societies have created ways and means of mitigating tensions—a holy river for ablution of the sin or a simple ritual to atone for a mistake or some ceremonies or counselling to cure a bleeding mind or a sense of atoning for the mistakes as a kind of pardoning oneself and so on. Prefer such sensual and social remedies involving movement of body, singing loudly with groups of friends, etc. if peace of mind is at stake. But never take to alcohol, wine, liquor, drugs like opium, cocaine, etc., even though it is tempting to find solace in it.

Try to come up in life. Never be jealous of those who have come up by hard work. Plan for a better future, rather than wasting time by yielding to thoughts of jealousy or envy. In life, one cannot wear the shoes of someone else and tread their path. Follow your path, even if it is simple and less productive. God has not created all as equals, but has destined all to play different roles.

Save at least 10 per cent of your earnings for future uncertainties. Keep yourself healthy. If possible, spend some of your earnings to help the unfortunate. If possible, help those within your circle who need help.

Keep yourself healthy by eating a variety of food and by maintaining your body neatly to avoid worries related to health.

Of course, none is perfect, and everyone falters in different stages, in different places, and in different times. Be empathetic within your means and capability while dealing with others. That will keep your mind to be in peace and tranquillity. Who knows, anyone may be in the same position, including me and you yourself, tomorrow.

LOOPING THOUGHTS

There are occasions when thoughts and worries revolve around themselves but never escape from the mind. The mind is completely immersed in thoughts and worries that the real world will be forgotten.

A person caught in the loop of tension and worries is lost in quicksand unless he comes out quickly. Sometimes, the person concerned may develop psychological problems due to looping worries, particularly if he loses sleep.

Looping thoughts about the opposite sex, particularly during adolescence, may affect the future very much.

The only way to come out of looping thoughts is through strong sensual impulse—it may be a pinch or loud sound or hunger and the like. So just like any good social animal, have the company of good friends and acquaintances and avoid loneliness.

Singing loudly may help to keep away looping thoughts and worries. Playing games with friends diverts the mind fully from worries. Physical work which does not need much mental concentration also relieves the looping thoughts. Also, talking to a friend or someone else on any non-controversial topic other than the looping worries will reduce the tension and help to come out of the loop and divert the mind.

Travel will give a lot of relief to come out of looping worries. Avoid driving since the chance for accidents is more.

If the looping tension is due to conscience, avoid past mistakes and try to help those who are affected by you, if possible. It is better to accept the mistake done in an honourable way rather than being haunted by it always.

MAINTENANCE OF THE MIND

Humans have a body with a mind integrated into it just like software is integrated with hardware for the proper functioning of a computer.

Humans are social animals and avoid lonely life. Ensure that you become a responsible member of the society. Check whether your conscience is in consonance with the ethical standards of the society. If the morals and ethics of the society prick your conscience, never hesitate to work for a change. But keep in mind that many social reformers and great philosophers failed in their attempt during their life time and many, including Socrates, Jesus Christ, etc., were victims of persecution by dogmatic, and influential, persons.

Behave with others the way you expect others to behave with you. Never think that all should maintain minimum etiquette while you feel that you can flout it. Also, a humane approach while dealing with others and their problems keeps the conscience clear.

Speech is as important as your behaviour. Never utter a word which would spoil the feeling of others unless warranted- but never try to please a criminal. The word that you utter and the word that comes in response to your word may hover together in the mind for days. A spilt word cannot be taken back.

You may do, as you think, no mistakes. But all are not like you. So have a maturity of mind to behave in a dignified way with those who do mistakes unknowingly.

To err is human. But ensure that the mistakes are within the limit of tolerance, and do not become blunders in life. Do not do anything which would haunt you later in the form of conscience, bad friends, etc. and whirl around past events. Moral values associated with societies differ from society to society, and one has to conduct oneself, as far as possible, according to the values associated with the society.

If one lives at the expense of others without doing any work when one is capable of doing some work, one becomes morally inferior and the mind becomes upset. So prefer to work and live with dignity rather than living on alms and charity forever. Do not dream of lottery or believe in gambling. That money is someone else's.

Try to save a little bit for future uncertainties or future investments. Never try to live on borrowed money. In particular, never borrow money for enjoying life.

Just like the changing seasons, happiness and sorrow, comfort and difficulties, peace of mind and tension, etc. are part of life, and they last for some time in each one's life. So when you are blessed with an abundance of happiness, money, etc., earn the goodwill of those associated with you like friends and relatives who would be pleased to help you when you are in trouble.

Remember that you are not standing alone and there is a web of people and invisible relations around you. There is a family, a society, a company or a place of work, a country, and a world with each one expecting something from you. Try to play the required role diligently.

Never be intoxicated by the abundance of happiness, comfort, etc. at any moment. Conduct yourself properly.

Sleep soothes the mind, and a normal adult needs eight to ten hours of sleep daily. For old persons who do not do any physical work, slightly less sleep may be sufficient. Children need ten to twelve hours of sleep daily. Lack of sleep charges the mind, and a charged mind does not do anything properly, particularly any mental work or minute physical work. Mistakes in the work or working for long hours to do a small work are the common problems associated with lack of sleep. Also, lack of sleep causes irritable behaviour- both for children and adults.

ANGER

Showing one's anger is not good in general, but not showing one's anger when needed may be dangerous.

While being angry, remember that all people do not think alike, and the capacity to do work, particularly perfect work, differs from person to person. Without proper briefing or understanding, each person tries to do work as he pleases or as he perceives or behaves in a manner that one likes.

By being angry, can you change the nature of the work done or the behaviour of a person? If the answer is *no*, never try to be angry, for it will produce no result except raising your blood pressure. In that case, try to accept the situation or condition of the work as it is without showing anger, or try to convince the concerned person without showing anger. Instead, showing anger may cause more serious mistakes out of panic.

Showing one's anger to solve the behavioural problems of children may be counterproductive in the long run. Repeated counselling, particularly when they are calm and receptive, may produce good results. Prefer to counsel them while they are eating or while they are in a receptive mood.

Also, frequently showing one's anger, even if it produces the desired result, is not good either for the person who shows anger or for the person who is shown the anger.

Remember that only a person who never bothers for the welfare or betterment of an institution, a family, or an individual may never show anger on anyone even if everything goes wrong.

One should protect oneself from one's own anger, failing which that anger will kill the person concerned.[36]

People who expect perfection in any work or those who are running short of time in doing their work are more likely to show anger frequently, which is likely to cause high blood pressure and other associated problems.

---

[36] Thirukkural: An ancient book containing 1,330 couplets in Tamil, a South Indian language.

FEAR

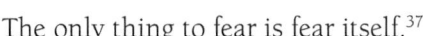

The only thing to fear is fear itself.[37]

The humans have the fear of the known as well as unknown—from the known snakes to unknown spirits.

The fear of punishment works so well that many social reformers used the fear of god to condition people to do what is good for the society and avoid what is bad. The fear of death was used for conditioning people not to do what the society forbids—it may be bad manners or immoral behaviour.

To bring accountability to one's conduct and behaviour in life, the fear of death was intertwined with the concept of hell after death. As the fear of death decreases with the advancement of science, the fear of hell decreases and one forgets one's accountability to one's actions and behaviour, forgetting that the Day of Judgement is ahead.

The fear of failure is so humiliating, and sometimes so catastrophic that sometimes people are prepared to win at any cost.

The fear of an unknown person, an unexplored place, etc. are so great that, till there is first-hand experience, one is ready to believe in rumours or imaginations based on piecemeal information.

---

[37] Franklin D. Roosevelt, an American president.

LOVE

Loving a person means giving the best of one's possession without expecting a return even if the return may be a natural outcome of the selfless giving. Unlike liking a material object or item, love has its psychological inscription.

If anyone likes someone and gives the best of the things, expecting something precious in return, then it can be termed not as love but as a smart business.

Love in a family will be sustained when love is mutual and the material and services are used for the welfare of the family and not to please the members of the family. If the materials and services are used only for pleasing the members of the family, the family has to face problems later. True love cannot put loved ones in problems and search for ad hoc solutions later.

Love is a filler of vacuum in the mind and is a psychological need for proper maintenance of the mind.

Love–hate relationships are inevitable in the society since the physical and psychological needs of a person transgress the needs of someone else in the society just like the needs of a sheep and a fox. One has to keep away from a hate relationship since it creates more psychological vacuum on one side of the mind and hence, psychological imbalance of the mind.

It is treacherous to pretend to be in love in a family. Love is an expression of inner feelings and not a shower of platitudes. Be truthful, for we get back what we give in life.

Love, like all emotions, does not follow any logic or reason. So an accidental love may change one's course in life completely. Teenage love may affect the studies of students very much.

Love should be felt by the deeds and behaviour and not through spoken words.

HAPPINESS

Happiness is an excited state of mind which gives a sense of psychological well-being. A person who is content in living within one's means and saves a little for future uncertainties is more happy compared to a person with an insatiable desire.

Happiness may also be related to sensual needs. One may be happy because of a tasty food; another may go mad after a lovely music; someone may enjoy good scenery in a mountain; someone else may find bliss in the company of his loved ones; etc.

Happiness is also a social need. A happy person is more sociable. A person may be more happy in social gatherings like talking to one's friends or enjoying with family members or playing a game with people in the locality or revelling in a festival and so on. Even though everyone is happy in one's own achievement, one is more happy when the achievement is recognized by the family, friends, or the society. A few appreciative words, a function recognizing an achievement, etc. bring more joy. A happy person can do more productive work in time.

Since there is no visible or measurable boundary for happiness, people tread beyond the limit, affecting the mind, body, and society. People found bliss in liquor affecting the body and mind to forget the world of pain and sorrow.

Craving for more happiness, people found asylum under drugs like cocaine, heroin, opium, etc. Psychologically, many became slaves of happiness and became addicted to drugs, never to come back to the real world of toil and pain. They die as physical and psychological wrecks. Strangely enough, people are ready to die for happiness or the promise of everlasting happiness in heaven after death. That is, the body and mind are in different worlds which are quite unrelated.

Happiness is a part of our life, and in pursuit of everlasting happiness, never spoil your body and mind. Life is a mixture of pain and pleasure, and everlasting happiness is just a mirage in life.

Money may help to bring happiness but money is not the only thing which brings happiness.

TRUTH AND THE NAKED TRUTH

Who wants to tell lies? Of course, none. But the cost of truth may be so high that most people may prefer not to tell it, some may prefer not to tell it for some time, some may mix it with lie, and a person with a conscience may dare to tell to a few.

However, this world survives since most of the people prefer to tell the truth as they perceive it even though their perceptions may differ or their perceptions may be contrary to the truth itself. When we see the sun moves around the earth, how to believe that the earth revolves around the sun?

Of course, truth triumphs. But truth triumphs alone at the fag end, leaving behind pain, misery, sufferings, perverted truth, and lies.

Truth is dressed in different vests and is interpreted according to the state of mind of the person. After being interpreted by different persons, what would be considered as truth may be far away from the truth.

Each person has a strength and weakness. The exposure of the truth about one's strength and weakness may become dangerous to the ego or even to the existence of the person.

A violent incident cannot be told to a child, or a horrible scene cannot be shown to a child. It has to be clothed with different coloured vests so that decency and mental acceptability is maintained. A lost battle may be told to the countrymen as a victory to keep the morale high, a mother may tell about the death of a grandfather to a child that he has gone to heaven or to a faraway place, a leader assures of final victory during war in spite of many debacles; a humiliating argument before the public is told to the spouse as the ignorance of the rules by the people, etc. Truth cannot always be told as it is to all. When people see a person in light, they ignore the shadow behind him and vice versa.

Socrates[38] proved the oracle of Delphi and exposed the ignorance of the rich, the powerful, and the sophists who pretended to be wise men. His exposure of the naked truth had cost him his life when the rich and the powerful people ganged against him and sentenced him to death.

It may need time or mental maturity to accept the naked truth. So share the naked truth with trusted and right people only in right time.

---

[38] The oracle of Delphi told that Socrates, an ancient Greek philosopher, was the wisest man on the earth. Socrates exposed those who claimed to be wise through rational arguments and logical conclusions. That made him enemies of many powerful persons, and he was accused of spoiling the minds of the youths of Athens. He was convicted to death and took hemlock, a kind of poison, and died.

ABSOLUTE TRUTH

Ideal place is nowhere in this world. So an ideal person hardly exists—even if an ideal person exists, it is against all odds or it is only for a brief time only.

Truth—absolute truth—exists briefly, for there is no ideal environment perpetually. Each one has his own reason to hide, or pervert, the truth so that his immediate or long term necessities are fulfilled.

Since man is born with ignorance and imperfection in an imperfect world with an instinct to survive, everyone has to hide his weakness so as to avoid being exploited by vested interests and other selfish people. Each one has to project his strength to get recognition and social status in the society. So most of the time, when the stakes are high, the truth is coloured or projected in such a way that even a believer starts doubting his own perception of truth.

Since no man is complete in all respects, there are always singularities in the form of absolute truth in a smooth life which, if exposed, may turn out to be Achilles' heel.[39]

---

[39]   Greek mythology: Achilles was the son of a sea nymph and a king. To make him immortal, his mother dipped him in the holy river Styx by holding him by the heels. Since his heels were not dipped in the holy river, his heels were the weakest point in his whole body. He was killed by an arrow striking his heel.

BRANCHES IN LIFE

Within the span of birth and death, the path each one treads is different. People like to do what they can understand or what brings happiness to them. 'What is simple' is understandable. Satisfaction of the senses of the body brings happiness.

In the long journey of life, men and women easily get diverted since their mind flows where they could do things which they can understand or where they could find happiness.

There are many things in life which distract the mind from following a path. Yes, there are a variety of lights, sounds, textures, and associated dreams that fascinate men and women which change their way of living forever. It may be beauty, money, strength, sweet words, big bungalow, etc.

Most of the diversions in life are accidental. A small incident in the house or school, a friend's advice, a deed by a hero in a film, etc. may change someone's life forever.

The normal diversion in life is the opposite sex. But when the diversion occurs during adolescence or before men and women are matured enough to live together, the effect of the diversion on life is tremendous.

Playing and enjoying in life is another diversion, and the mind flows towards it unhindered. The company of bad friends is a big diversion which affects life beyond remedy.

Necessity, willpower, resources, and the capability to surmount difficulties help to pursue higher aspirations or aims without branching. Listening to advice from proper persons will help to reduce the problems while moving without branching.

The biggest effect of diversion in life is the waste of time. Without realizing the short span of life, one gets too old to achieve anything.

MANIFESTATION OF TRUTH IN LIFE

Truth manifests in life but never governs life since everyone is born selfish with an instinct to survive.

In life, the physical and psychological encounters that one experiences are unique on the whole that each one realizes something unique before death. A greedy man realizes that he has to leave all his wealth. A kind mother realizes that she has to leave her lovely children. A rich person realizes that he should have looked after his health also. An old person realizes that each one should have saved some money while young, for old-age emergencies. A monk realizes that everyone should die even if he is the beloved son of god. A disciplinarian realizes that too much discipline spoils the atmosphere in life. A beautiful lady realizes that her beauty fades away slowly. A successful person realizes that failures are part of life. An honest person realizes that honesty does not always produce the desired result. A criminal realizes what he did was against the norm of humanity. An educated man realizes that his education did not teach him the essence of life. A selfish person realizes that life means more than survival. A rich man realizes that bringing up children with tasty food is not enough in life. A priest realizes that flattery and rituals are not enough to please a god. A food fiend realizes that life means more than tasty food and beautiful bodies. A religious fanatic realizes that people of other religions also survive and flourish, most probably with the blessings of his own supreme god! In the course of one's life, a perfectionist realizes that she has no choice but to live the life with its own twists and turns and not according to her plan. A drunkard realizes that liquor has moth-eaten more of his life than his enjoyment of liquor.

What is life? Is there any purpose of living? Is life just survival? Is life for eating and merrymaking only? Just like any animal, everyone is selfish. So shall we survive anyhow at others' expenses? Just like the parents who prepare their children for living their life, is there anyone who prepares to face death? Is there any meaning in living one's life? Do life and death have any significance in life?

Since we get back what we give in life, not necessarily in terms of money, comfort, etc., each one realizes the attributes of life and their significance in life in a different way. None realizes life in its entirety. In the life tree, each one branches in time to experience the truth through the twisted branches of the tree and not through the whole tree. The whole truth about life is incomprehensible since most attributes have less relevance to one's experiences in life.

EXCEPTIONS OR SINGULARITIES

Every rule has an exception in nature and some of the rules, on many occasions.

What was thought to be a smooth curve in life may end in a singularity with an unimaginable speed and unpredictable consequences. The singularity may be a break or an unreachable height or an unfathomable depth. What was thought to be predictable becomes unpredictable sometimes. What was seen as a calm and serene sea creates a storm threatening the life and livelihood of many. A calm and quiet earth shivers in the form of an earth quake.

In the time–life curve, every curve has many singularities pushing many to this and that side and chartering unplanned courses in life. The singularities give a lesson for the future or a turning point for a better life or a welcome respite from pain and sufferings.

The handling of exceptions or singularities changes a good person into a rogue or a bad person to repent throughout life. The change that the exceptions or singularities bring in life may be physical or psychological.

Exceptions or singularities give a message that there is something which is beyond one's control and which one failed to learn or understand. Without exceptions or singularities in one's life, man will assert himself a god—a man who is born to achieve everything he wants.

The rise or fall created by exceptions or singularities in life is sudden and unpredictable. Hence, behave well during the happy days so that there is someone to lift you up when fallen.

BOUNDARY

There is a boundary for everything in life within which the concerned thing works and beyond which it loses its effect. Remember, a mighty lion is powerless in water while a crocodile becomes invincible in water. A mighty king has his power within his own country. Even a mighty bomb has its own limit by destroying nearby objects only. The teachings of a wise man may be liked by a few people with a conscience while the majority fear that their source of enjoyment will be lost. The desires of kings to expand their kingdoms were met with stiff opposition that limited the boundary of their kingdoms.

A popular beautiful person in a society may not be accepted as beautiful in some other society. The richest person in a country may not be able to buy a small piece of land in some other country. All comfort, food, and money may not be able to buy a child from a poor mother. The president of a powerful country may be helpless in keeping a protester silent.

The power of a parent to direct a child to do certain things is up to a certain age or a certain time only. The power of a person to impose one's will on the spouse is subject to the consent of the spouse. The joy of being with one's family in a pleasant tourist spot may be limited to a few days only. Bearing the tyranny of a teacher may be only for a few years for a child.

The desire of a person to become more and more rich has its own limit resulting in an invisible boundary. The desire of a scholar to know more and more is limited to an invisible boundary. The desire of a person to harm his enemy is limited in reality. Even truth may have its own boundary for establishing truth while there is a bone of contention.

SPACE FOR NEEDS

As far as the needs of life are concerned, none is endowed with everything one needs or cherishes always. At any time, a few needs may be satisfied in abundance while a few other essential needs diminish within the space for life.

Needs within the Space for Life at Any Time

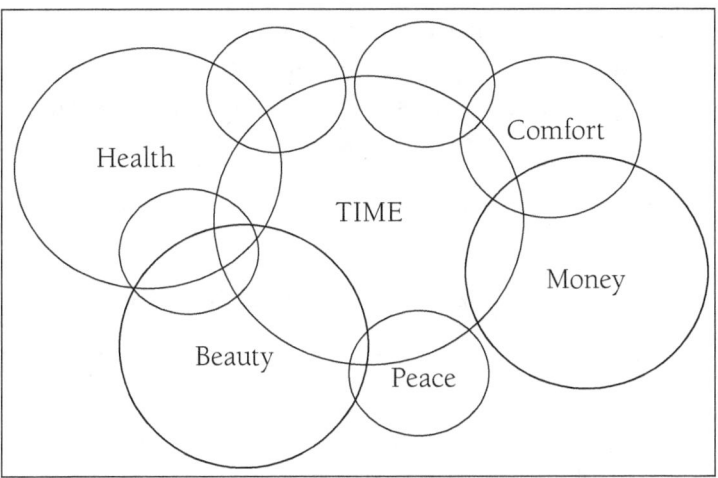

When one has a lot of time, money, etc., some other requirements get diminished automatically. One may be busy with time, but he may not have the time to enjoy life and comfort; one may have a lot of time but she may have no money; one may have a lot of money, but the health may not be all right; one might have achieved a feat, but it might have cost a lot of time—years of training and preparation; one may have all types of comfort, but there may be no peace of mind; one may be happy, but he may not have more money; one may be honest, but there may be no recognition of his honesty; one may have beauty, but she may not have enough money; and so on.

In short, the physical and psychological needs of each one of us adjust themselves within the space of life. 'Everything for everyone at every time' is an unrealizable goal in life; if it becomes true, life becomes static and the rein of heaven dawns for all.

If there is abundance of one resource expanding within the life–space diagram for a person, then there is a shortage of another resource, leading to a shrinking in life space since the space to accommodate it is less within the life–space diagram, as explained in the Venn diagram.

FEELINGS AND ATTITUDE

The feelings and attitude towards a person can expand or constrict within the space according to one's perception about the person and the environment in which both are there at a time.

Space for Feelings within the Mind

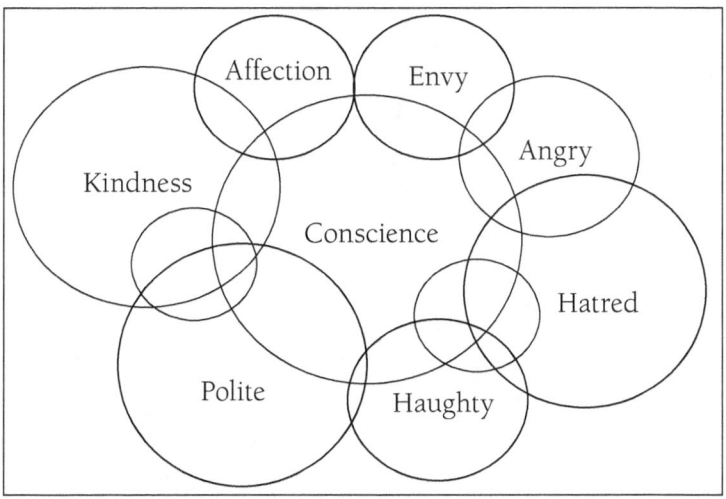

When hatred expands in one's mind, kindness, empathy, politeness, etc. shrink to accommodate hatred. An angry person hardly finds any polite word. A happy heart hardly has any space for envy at any moment. A compassionate person hardly finds any place for hatred. A greedy person hardly shows any sympathy towards a poor person.

Of course, the conscience pricks when one's harsh words or deeds hurt another person and one experiences a similar situation later. The heart of the Good Samaritan was filled with kindness, empathy, etc. when he saw a helpless man.

VIOLENCE AND NON-VIOLENCE

Violence is not the only law in a jungle. If a deer fears a lion, then the flies and mosquitoes are a menace to the lion with which it has to live with. The might of the lion has no power over the flies and mosquitoes. If violence or might is the law of the jungle on a few occasions, it is also a law of the civil society sometimes. Violence exists in different forms, from a local thug to a powerful army. Non-violence and the rule of reason or law also exist in all societies depending on the social maturity based on the social evolution of the society.

Violence and non-violence coexist in society. If war and peace is for the society, then violence and non-violence is for an individual. Violence exists in different forms, including the threat of violence. Unchallenged violence leads to criminalisation of the society.

Corruption, bad behaviour, unreasonable demands, etc. lead to challenging of the person concerned which leads to violence when the concerned person does not see reason. If challenging a criminal element with a violent motive is treated as violence, then no civil society can survive.

Had not Hitler unleashed violence and waged war, many women in the society might not have dreamt of equality. Men went to the war front which led to the shortage of manpower during World War II. That helped women get employment in many fields which were the monopoly of men only. Also, African- Americans in the USA got some job opportunities.

If human civilisations are the victims of violence, then many a noble soul are also the victims of violence which retards the social progress in many societies. Non-violence and the reasonable rule of law lead to a variety of development, peace, and progress. Of course, *in peace, there is progress.*[40]

Violence sprouts from the mind. As in a jungle, the physical and psychological impact of violence is so great that none dares to challenge it, and society has adjusted itself to violence as a way of life throughout the world.

Preaching non-violence to criminal elements is nothing but cowardice on the part of the society and individuals. Injustices, cheating, betrayal of trust, unquestionable power in one's hands, skewed wealth in one's hands, etc. lead to violence in the society.

Non-violence is a tool of protest only in a civilized society. Instead of British rule, had Mahatma Gandhi led his civil disobedience movement under an autocrat like Hitler, there may be no Mahatma Gandhi[41] at all.

---

[40]   *In his book on World War II, Sir* Winston Churchill, Prime Minister of England during World War II writes that in 'peace - *progress'.*

[41]   Mohandas Karamchand Gandhi, who led India to independence from British rule through non-violence.

MAN IN THE SOCIETY

Man is a social animal, and his success in survival is due to his cooperative social living.

Man is born free, and everywhere he is in chains, as observed by Jean-Jacques Rousseau[42].

The invisible rules in the family in the form of conduct and behaviour, the rules of the society in the form of customs and traditions, and the laws of the land where one is born, are binding and set limitations to one's freedom and equality.

In spite of the limitations and boundaries set by the family and the society, man is a social animal and prefers to live in the society which gives protection as well as a means of livelihood besides a sense of psychological well-being.

A lonely person without a social life is likely to form extreme views which may be positive or negative.

The advantages of living in a society are greater. With each one being born selfish, only an acceptable behaviour assuring personal safety and the safety of the property of the members in the society is essential, which limits the freedom of an individual to do anything one likes to do. Only an enlightened society with a liberal outlook can

---

[42]   A French Philosopher whose work 'Social Contract' was also one of the causes for French Revolution.

ensure freedom, particularly the freedom of conscience and the freedom from fear.

Societies which were formed from close-knit families collapsed due to a mutually agreed existence or submission to violence. Primitive societies which were formed in the name of the laws of god collapsed in the course of time because of the effort of great thinkers and social reformers who dared death to challenge the inhuman laws of the society.

Social life is an important aspect in one's life, with each member in the society observing certain norms in one's conduct and behaviour, particularly with juniors, with equals, and with elders.

Good manners are essential prerequisites for social interactions in a society. Good manners are just introductory in the interactions with the members of the society, and their effect is limited if the time of interaction with the members of the society is long. As time increases, the need, interest, and behaviour of the persons affect the interactions.

Good societies provide free public spaces for social gatherings, playing, social activities, reading, etc.

MANAGEMENT

Strangely enough, most of the world's successful managers are people of average calibre. In general, the world is managed successfully at all levels, except at the micro level, by average people. This is evident in the management from a family to a country.

The micro level is managed by experts in the relevant field, whereas a manager monitors the overall outcome of each or almost all micro-level work for the successful integration of the work.

Even if a manager is average or below average, a good manager always listens to experts or good advisors before deciding the course of action.

A manager, who plans by consulting all concerned and distributes work to the right persons and briefs them properly, will succeed in doing the work. A good manager judges the capability, needs, and nature of his employees and assigns the work accordingly. Treating all the employees as equals hardly works.

But a manager who does not monitor or pretend to monitor his employees hardly achieves his target even if all the employees are good.

It is the management of the personnel which is very delicate. A manager who does not listen to the personal problems being faced by his employees and does not try to help whenever possible can hardly expect that his employees will wholeheartedly help for the success of the task assigned at a crucial juncture.

EQUALITY

At any moment in this world, there is no equality in the society as far as the physical and psychological needs are concerned. And so life flows. The potentials and efforts of each person in different attributes of life are so different that two persons cannot be made equal at any time. The potentials of the different attributes of life are not stable, and the changes are dynamic. It is the greatness of the human heart to accept that all are equal in the society at all times.

Inequality is everywhere in a glaring manner. One is born to a rich person while another is poor; one is strong while another is weak; one is intelligent while another is ready to do only what is ordered; one is honest while another person is waiting for a chance to cheat; one is white in complexion while another is black; one wishes to work and live while another finds pleasure in living on others' earnings; one produces food for the society while another sings a song for the society; one prepares food while another prepares implements for preparing food; and so on.

In some societies, inequality was institutionalized in the name of god. Women were ill-treated, and men were humiliated in the name of god[43], as in Hinduism. At least some gods were more humane, as in Buddhism, Christianity, Sikhism, etc., and accepted all men as equal, whereas most of the primitive gods had a hierarchical status among themselves just like the rich and powerful in this world, and hence, their devotees were stratified and treated as inferiors or superiors in the society. Slavery and colonialism created high-class and low-class societies. Vested interests and privileged classes suppressed revolts for equality through violence and treachery, as was the fate of Buddhism in India.

At a time when people were ready to die for honour and privileges and when there was no substitute for a king, the signing of Magna Carta[44] created a sense of equality

---

[43] Rig Veda, an ancient Sanskrit literature in India, divides the society into four divisions called varnas. They are divided based on birth. It was claimed that Brahma, the god of Birth, creates man from different parts of his body. A man born from the head of Brahma becomes a Brahman (priest), the highest varna; if born from the chest, he becomes a Kshatriya (warrior); if born from the stomach, he becomes a Vaisya (businessman); and if born from the legs, he becomes a Sudra (worker), the lowest varna. Women do not belong to any varna. Varna is hereditary, and it cannot change. Each varna became innumerable castes later, and vested interests exploited the society in the name of caste and god.
Manusmriti, a criminal code of conduct for Hindus, sets different rules and punishments for each varna and ill-treats all lower varnas. The lower the Varna, the higher the punishment will be for the same crime.

[44] Magna Carta forced King John to accept rules and laws for governance as far as the barons (feudal lords) were concerned, and the barons should extend the feudal concessions to their tenants (subjects).

among King John of England and his barons. In the course of time, it led to a morally egalitarian society in England and a democratic constitution.

Even though inequality is everywhere and the society accepted it as a fait accompli, the French Revolution against the king and nobles, the Russian Revolution for social equality, and to some extent, the American War of Independence forcefully spread the message of equality. Books and mass communication made it easier to spread the idea of equality. Because of equality, snobbery started disappearing, and courteous behaviour was expected from all.

World wars made things easier for those who yearned for equality. All men were needed to fight the enemy besides the elite who were trained to fight and paid dearly. Even women, the undeclared slaves of men in each society, were given employment which was a source of financial independence from the shackles of dependence, and a sense of equality spread in the society.

Even though kings and royals have disappeared from the scene, many, particularly those in power, enjoy power and privileges for the smooth performance of their administrative duties. With flatterers and sycophants surrounding them, the people in power become despots, and equality disappears. Institutions set up to protect equality were forced to be mere helpless spectators.

LIBERTY

A free man is chaotic, and if everyone is free to do what one likes, then none can live in peace in a society. So each society framed its own rules and regulations for its members to follow and monitored them through social and religious institutions. Man is born free, but his freedom is restricted for the welfare of the society.

A free man in a natural state has to fight for existence with others, for each one is selfish. If the members of the society are not equal before the social institutions, then rules and laws made for each stratum of the society differ. So the liberty and the privileges associated with the liberty varied for each stratum of the society.

In some societies, goons and thugs threaten the society and subvert liberty where the social institutions are weak or when they are manned by unfit men. '... where there is no law there is no freedom; for liberty is to be free from restraint and violence from others, which cannot be where there is no law; ...'[45] So when unfit people administer social institutions, personal or social liberty is suppressed due to poor management of law and order till a social evolution or revolution takes place.

---

[45] John Locke, a British philosopher.(Source: Social Contract Locke-Hume-Rousseau, with introduction by Sir Ernest Barker)

ROLE PLAY

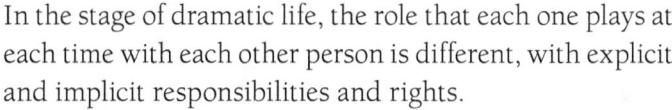

In the stage of dramatic life, the role that each one plays at each time with each other person is different, with explicit and implicit responsibilities and rights.

A person can play the role of a father or a mother, a son or a daughter, a servant or a master, a king or a clown, an officer or an employee, etc. with the associated privileges and responsibilities of each role.

With each role that one plays, the implicit range of influence of the role is determined, affecting many lives and the environment within an implicit boundary.

While a teacher can influence a few hundred students, a father or a mother can influence a few in the family. A leader can influence a country, a reformer can influence a community, and a thinker or philosopher can influence the whole world.

With different roles being played by the same person at different times and with different rights and responsibilities associated with each role, as the range of influence increases, the power and responsibility increases tremendously as is the case of a minister, mayor of a city, etc.

As the range of influence increases, the implicit and explicit bonds that regulate the individual's thinking and movement become weakened, and one can observe random irregular movements which are not related to the range of influence.

So play your role responsibly so that those who move ahead with the light you are showing do not face any problem in following the path trodden by you or shown by you.

LONELINESS

Man being a social animal, loneliness is anathema to the society. Loneliness creates opinions, thoughts, and dogmas which may be logically or emotionally incorrect. But the views of a lonely person cannot be corrected if wrong and cannot be implemented in the society if right.

Once views or dogmas are formed based on bitter experiences in the home or society, loneliness breeds extreme views which may be dangerous for the person as well as the society.

Each society devised its own way of bringing all people into its fold by organizing festivals, rituals, pilgrimages, etc. with relatives and others periodically.

The emotional attachment created on face-to-face contact, with each one speaking freely what is in the mind and helping others in a small way, brings a sense of belongingness.

As parents grow old, it is the loneliness which would be haunting them. Grandchildren reduce the loneliness of grandparents. Also, children break the looping thoughts and tensions arising out of loneliness.

Those who are haunted by loneliness may find some hobbies to do, some books to read, some creative work to do, some social service to do, a tour to travel, etc.

EXTREMISM

The safe way in life is to tread the middle path, but near the extremes and boundaries and away from the middle path, the rules and principles governing an individual and society are unenforceably weak and questioned. Every rule has an exception depending on the time, place, person, etc., and so there are a few who differ from the majority on many occasions.

As the middle path is comfortable for many, the ideals and principles with the associated rituals are converted into dogma.

With the changing time and with new experience, perception of the rules and principles governing the dogma change, particularly for those off the middle path. But when the dogma is enforced by the majority through threat and violence, the extremism of the majority results in the meek submission or psychological slavery of the minority.

When views and ideals become dogmatic, the only alternative to free oneself from unrealistic and meaningless life is extremism. When there is no person or system to address the grievances and when dissent or protest does not lead to any fruitful result, the alternative would be meek submission or a revolt. Extremism of the minority is associated with revolt, and a charged atmosphere prevails in both camps—followers of normal customary views or extreme views. Sometimes, extremism of the minority results in the exploitation of the majority, and there comes a situation when the majority is not ready to yield to the bullies of the minority. Naturally, it leads to a kind of showdown.

Remember that non-violence is one of the ways to tackle extremism, but it works only in a civilized society where responsible people are ready to listen, think, and make necessary changes.

When views become dogmatic, thinking becomes unreasonable due to the changed environment, and the living environment becomes intolerable and hostile. Then extremism springs up in the family or in the society.

Moderation of extreme views is possible only when people come closer, exchange their views in an amicable atmosphere, and accept a reasonable interpretation of rituals, behaviours, ideas, rules, etc.

Nature and history has shown that extremism is a random phenomenon in all societies, bringing out some changes in their philosophies and ideals.

Extremism explodes when reason surrenders before dogma or the selfishness of a few try to envelope the society.

SOCIAL REVOLUTION

Revolts and rebellions are common against established authority in the history of humans, but a revolution, which changes the authoritative set up of the society, as in the case of the French and Russian revolutions, is rare.

Each person in the society is normally adjustable and accommodative towards bullying, exploitation, etc. to some extent as long as it does not affect one's honourable living. Society is tolerant when the authority, like a king, is exploiting or not helpful in any way. 'Great mistakes in the ruling part, many wrong and inconvenient laws, and all slips of human frailty will be borne by the people without mutiny or murmur.'[46]

When the authority exploits society openly and deliberately for a long time and when it refuses to listen to the society when the society is in trouble, revolution takes place when there is no other means of finding a different way.

When the authority is reasonable and responsive, to some extent, to the demands of the society or when there are other means of changing the authority or controlling the authority, there is no question of revolution.

In a civilized society, there is no chance of revolution since there are avenues through which one can air one's

---

[46]   John Locke, a British philosopher.

grievances or challenge an authority, and there is a chance for change on either side.

God and religion are antidotes for revolution even in extreme circumstances since god gives hope for a better tomorrow.

An emotionally disagreeing person may revolt against an established authority in a family when there is no way of venting their feelings. So listen to the demands and longings of the family members patiently and yield to their petty demands occasionally, if necessary, under protest.

WAR AND PEACE

If the history of man is any indicator, man cannot live without war. From time immemorial, war-weary man longed for peace, and peace-weary man opted for war. War sprouts in the minds of man and slowly gathers into a storm. Man becomes excited and is not amenable to reason when victory can be achieved with fewer casualties or if it can inflict more damages on the enemy. A small incident, which is the culmination of a series of unacceptable happenings, becomes an excuse to start a war, and the war or its effect drags on for a long time, exciting the minds of the victorious and inciting the minds of the humbled. Just like the electric charge that builds up in the clouds, slowly acquiring a specific charge, a surcharged mind is induced with a series of accidental or planned incidents with peculiar justifications on both sides and coming to diametrically opposite conclusions. And war follows till both sides come to know that it cannot be won without suffering heavy losses inflicted by the opposite side.

No selfish person can live without quarrels, explicit or implicit, and no selfish nation can live without war, explicit or implicit. A selfish leader can create a selfish nation by giving a promise of plenty or promising to subdue a monster which is likely to threaten the survival of the nation.

In a surcharged atmosphere, the loud voice of the value of peace or the cost of war or the simple logic or reason is neither heard by a clever leader nor liked by his followers.

It may be easy to live with an honest enemy, but very difficult to live with criminal elements. It is much more honourable to go to war rather than buy peace with criminal elements. Peace cannot be bought, but it has to be earned by both sides by their reasonable conduct and diplomacy, and not by bullying or appeasing.

WAR

Just like singularities faced by individuals, in the life of countries, there are events which change the history, mostly due to war.

It is human to fight for survival, just like any other animal. Man is born selfish, and, as ordained by gods and society, to keep one's own society safe from other societies, he never hesitates to fight, particularly when he sees more wealth to loot or more authority to assert over others, if he wins the war.

Just like each one in a society, each country in this world is interdependent. Each country needs the resources of other countries, like men, material, and other products and services. No country is endowed with all that is needed for it—it may be food or materials or men to do menial work or skilled work and the like.

Denial or scarcity makes the scrambling to get the resources anyhow. A country which is deprived of the needed resources from another country on its own terms and conditions may find an excuse, in connivance with other countries inimical to the latter, to go for war, particularly when it can win with the least damage. When the enemy can inflict considerable damage, there may be an attempt to bully, and propaganda wars may start to justify threatening speeches, but the chance for war is less.

Also, man is selfish, and a selfish leader may exploit the selfishness of their countrymen to go for war and loot the resources of another country.

Also, a government in trouble may prefer a war to divert the attention of its people.

For each country, its national interest is paramount. That is, selfishness is paramount compared to the natural law of reason and justice for all. With no accepted system or organization like the British system of legislature, executive, judiciary and an appellate body to govern or to redress the grievances of all countries, it is not possible to avert another war. Countries which are incapable of defending themselves are likely to be offended with impunity by powerful nations in any war even if the war is not related to them.

As disagreement leads to animosity, the 'gathering of storm'[47] of war is inevitable as history replays its drama again.

But countries having more power and privileges hardly give them up in favour of a naturally equitable arrangement, and a few countries may stand up to the bullying by the powerful and the privileged, particularly when it affects their right to live an honourable life.

Man's instincts and thinking has not changed in the course of evolution, and so man's learning from history is always short-lived. Also, history has its own paradoxes, human fallacies, perverted truths, and veiled lies as well as absolute truths. History is told by the victors who had the privilege of lying under official secret acts. What are

---

[47]   Sir Winston Churchill, Prime Minister of England during World War II, describes the events prelude to World War II thus.

the causes of events leading to the present history? The future generation can never know the mystery behind the causes of war since the real reason for war, as felt by the vanquished, will never be known, and so there is a real chance for repeating history. Was Hitler[48] always wrong? Was it possible to rally most of the Germans around Hitler on lies and falsehood alone? Of course, he gave self-respect to the Germans who had been forced to accept humiliating conditions by the victors after World War I. Countries enjoying privileges will never be ready to forego them even in unrealistic situations, and countries pushed to the wall due to harsh realities or logical deductions of history will prick the big fat bully in the course of time. So, future war is inevitable.

The possibility of war is more in the present scenario since there are special interest propaganda groups and special interest flatterers and sycophants around powerful persons. Greedy syndicates with vested interests in each country can influence the power centres in some countries to go to war or incite to go to war.

In spite of the huge cost of war in terms of lost lives or damaged properties, each war leaves a trail of some benefits to the other side of the society. If World War II were not fought, European women might not have got equal opportunity or employment, African-Americans in USA might not have got employment opportunities, many countries in Asia and Africa might not have got independence from European colonial powers, etc. So

---

[48] Hitler was the Chancellor of Germany during World War II. The Allied Powers—Britain, France, USA, and Russia—were fighting against the Axis Powers, Germany, Italy, and Japan.

man is also forced to learn from bitter wars but falls into amnesia to play the same role in history again.

Let us learn history, and if possible, learn true history to avoid the past conflict and horrors, but never ask for reparations from the descendants of the perpetrators of evil, for birth is an accidental creation of providence for many in a callous society. The past history cannot be re-enacted as per our will, but at least, the future course of all our life may steer away from the embers of the past. Kindling the past history may overshadow the future but forgetting the past history is equivalent to disowning the present. Learn history to avoid repetition of history.

Great civilisations were destroyed more by the moral decline of their leaders and their people than by the barbaric nature of their opponents, for both groups will not hesitate to destroy each other through violence for material benefit and comfort.

HELP

Only a person who needs help, but is helpless, knows the value of timely help. People from European countries offered help even to enemies who needed help such as shipwrecked seafarers.

All members of a society are interdependent, and each one needs others' help sometimes. A person who feels that he does not need anyone's help may become arrogant, and he may never try to help anyone. Such people prefer punishment for each mistake, retribution, or revenge for any wrongdoings, right to privilege for themselves, etc.

In small societies like villages where interdependence is more, help will come unsolicited. People believe in each other.

In big cities where no one depends on others except through regulated systems based on rules, money, power, etc., rarely anyone bothers to help others since none is directly dependent on others.

In big cities and towns, spontaneous help has become a kind of charity, and a person whose mind is broad enough to help others offers help. But on many occasions, even if anyone wants to help, one may not find time to help since each one is busy in their own work.

MONEY

Ever since man invented money and traded it in exchange for goods, money had become an essential part of each one's life. Since money can buy many things, money and comfort in life go together. So, man devised many ways to get money without hard work like gambling, raffle, etc. Looting gold and valuables from people of other societies (or from giants, as our fables say) and enriching oneself was accepted as god's gift by most societies.

Amassed wealth, if used properly, is a good source of investment for any person and the society.

Since there is no measurable or visible upper limit of money that one can have, the insatiable desire to have more and more money makes man greedy to the extent of looting or robbing others' money. Man is so greedy that a medicine costing a few pennies is sold for a year's earning of a patient! Blood suckers of the society will demand, and be given, concessions while a poor man's food will be taxed.

The value for money that each one puts on it is not the same. Based on the place, time, and person, the value for money varies. The value for hard-earned money is more, and one feels difficult to part with it without equivalent goods in exchange.

The value for easy money is less. So, more easy money, compared to a normal amount, will be spent for purchasing the same item or for doing any work. A person who works hard and becomes rich may hesitate to waste money, but his children may become extravagant since the money is easy money for them.

Since the lure of money can buy a false witness for a rich man or protect a sinner from justice or cause public resources to be diverted to a few rich persons, causing misery for many, and the like, the environment in which the rich people are living is different, and hence, many scriptures proclaimed that the rich are least likely to go to heaven even though most of the gods depend on the rich man's charity for their rituals and ceremonies.

But poverty attracts all vices. When a poor person needs money for some essential services and vicious forces are in the lookout for a prey, a poor person is defenceless against the vices, whereas a rich person can at least fight against them. So work hard to rise above poverty.

POWER

Power and responsibility go together. Power without responsibility makes an autocrat. Responsibility without power is meaningless. This includes paternal power also.

It is easy to oppose a good person even when he is right, but it is dangerous to oppose an evil person even if he is wrong. So autocrats continued to rule throughout the world till war or mass revolts like the French Revolution and the Russian Revolution changed the handlers of power.

Uncontrolled power always leads to an impression of absolute victory which further leads to a chain of events greatly affecting those close to the person concerned and the society.

Without power, there is no order in the society, and so, power has to be vested with someone trustworthy. Since man is fallible, '... to live by one man's will become the cause of all men's misery.'[49]

In Great Britain, starting from Magna Carta till today's parliamentary system, power-sharing evolved logically according to the situation of the time, and other countries adopted different systems. But whatever be the system, if the person managing the system is corrupt, he will

---

[49] Hooker as quoted by Sir Ernest Barker in his compilation *Social Contract: Essays by Locke, Hume, and Rousseau.*

find ways to misuse power and, at the same time, shield himself using the power.

A group can manage better than an individual taking care of different aspects of power and governance. In case of misuse of power, the chance of exposure is possible in most cases.

Power can bring wonderful changes in life, but unbridled power may result in unmanageable miseries for many.

Power is very powerful like a sword, but so light that one is tempted to swipe it and test it on those who are likely to offer the least resistance. Since power flows through the path of the least resistance, it can harm the innocent more than those who rise in revolt and oppose, if misused.

SEX WITH MONEY AND POWER

The influence of money and power together with the associated sex in a person's behaviour is immense. In the history of mankind, there were major changes due to the influence of the above.

By nature, none is endowed with all of them at the same time. The effort to achieve what one wants anyhow normally leads to dramatic consequences. The struggle to have enough money, power, and sex leads to an ordinary life in the society. But those who have either abundance of money or unbridled power indulge in sex which goes beyond the realm of modesty.

Since sex has its own limitation and power was with men, many humiliating rules were made for women in the name of god and tradition. When not attained within a reasonable time, sex may lead to serious mental imbalances and psychological trauma. It is better to consult a doctor. A good friend with a reasonable experience in life or a reasonable outlook may be able to help to overcome the psychological storm in the mind.

In a civilized society, the power of money, power, and sex cannot be underestimated. They can change the world order or change the outlook and behaviour of a person. Everyone needs them and in the right quantity. But strangely enough, none has them in an appropriate quantity, depending on the physical and psychological make-up of the person at any time. Life flows in search of other things having different potentials, physically and psychologically.

Misuse of money, power, and sex may bring catastrophes or disasters in life. Power without responsibility or money without utility or sex without fidelity is dangerous to the mental health of any person. Friends may desert or society may rise in anger or a spouse may live in the mental world of hell in this real world when money or power or sex is misused or misappropriated.

Sometimes, the risk of exposure of socially forbidden sex is so great that people go to any extent to hide it. Can anyone imagine that King Agamemnon, the victorious commander of the Trojan War would be killed by his own unfaithful wife?[50]

---

[50]   Greek mythology: After winning the Trojan War, Agamemnon, king of Mycenae, returned to his kingdom where his wife Clytemnestra killed him with assistance from her lover, Aegisthus.

ECOLOGY

This world is a participative world for all animals including humans, the last animal in the series of evolution.

Man's success in survival and proliferation of his progeny have made him to think that he is the owner of this world and all flora and fauna are only for his benefit and enjoyment. Man is inebriated with success in the race for survival that his kingdom started encroaching and destroying the kingdoms of most of the animals and plants.

The role of each plant and animal, including humans, is unique in the preservation of the environment. The change from partnership to ownership of the world has resulted in destroying anything for comfort or pleasure or vanity.

But man cannot survive alone. Man is dependent on plants and animals, and a nurturing environment which nourishes them.

Just like any animal, man is selfish, and without an enlightened selfishness, man may directly and indirectly destroy the nurturing environment of the flora and fauna which helps him to survive and flourish.

Just like any animal, man should learn to coexist with the plants and the animals, failing which man may become a prominent mammal in the list of the extinguished.

Do not scorn at spiders, lizards, frogs, etc. which help you kill disease-spreading mosquitoes and other insects. Allow them to live nearby, if possible.

Try to dispose of the waste properly. A piece of bone may be given to a dog; dirty water may be diverted to a tree; etc.

If man, as a victor, sets terms and conditions and starts encroaching the kingdoms of all flora and fauna, the effect would be bitter and devastating, which would be learnt as was learnt by the Allied forces in World War II which resulted because of the humiliating conditions imposed on the defeated Germany[51] after World War I.

---

[51] After World War I, the Treaty of Versailles forced Germany to lose all its colonies and some territories as reparations for war to the victors and to reduce the defence forces to a farce that it cannot defend Germany, etc. That was the source of World War II, causing more death and destruction.

JUDGEMENT IN LIFE

Just like the design of a ship is judged by how it survives the storms, one's life is judged by how one faces the difficult phases in life. No one is assured of a peaceful life forever since there are physical deprivations, accidents, psychological eruptions, sensual deprivations or social protests, and the like in life.

With success never guaranteed, how do we judge our lives? Even though we are born selfish, do we behave with others with enlightened selfishness which is needed in any society for cooperative living, or do we see only our own interest as the ultimate goal?

Do our dependants see us as masters who should be obeyed or as leaders who should be followed?

Do we see those who failed or who are helpless with empathy, or do we see ourselves as superiors or heroes?

Are the values cherished by one at variance with the normal human values? Do we see our views, behaviour, and conduct with a touchstone of conscience, or do we see through the prism of success alone?

In spite of the successes and failures that one experiences in life, a person is not judged by survival alone, but by the values that one cherishes and by the spirit with which one is ready to defend one's values and conducts oneself accordingly. The contribution by a person to the family or society may be small or big according to the position or power that one holds in the society or the environment in which one lives.

Are we enlightened enough that our judgement withstands the onslaught of time beyond our existence?

LIFE IN DIFFERENT COLOURS

Life can be described not in uniformity but in variety—in terms of different colours, just like a rainbow; in different speeds, like the speed of a snail and the speed of a leopard; in different mediums, like a bird in air or a fish in water; in different moods, like enjoying the fun or angry and intolerant; in different activities, like managing the house or managing a country; in different tastes, like eating sweets or tasting bitter medicines; in different types of enjoyment, like spending the time with children or enjoying an orchestra; etc.

The attributes of life—whether taste or mood or anything else—cannot be explained in specific words or shown in specific visuals. Just like Eve's[52] curiosity landed her in this world for tasting the sweetest apple in heaven, each person is curious to experience life and its variety within the constraints of each one's life. The young is tempted to experience the varieties of life and refuse to listen to the words of the experienced and enlightened wise persons. So life revolves in a cycle with the same phases being experienced by parents and children in different times—a father watches his son fall for the same

---

[52]   Bible: Eve and her companion, Adam, were forbidden by god to eat apples in the Garden of Eden. But Eve ate it out of curiosity, and Adam ate, not to miss the company of Eve. Both were thrown by god in this harsh world.

type of temptation that he fell on while he was young but realizes the implications later or a mother watches her daughter flying high with the same dreams as she had or a father watches helplessly as his sons fight against each other, just like sworn enemies, for getting more share of his property as the father fought with his brother for the prime property and so on.

Life has to be assessed in totality—the variety of deeds that one performs and the constraints under which they were done.

For shaping the life, one has to see the green and the red or taste the sweet and the sour or see the alluring beauty and the odd abstract figure or experience the cool bath in the summer and hiking over a mountain in winter and so on. Any attempt to shape life through a mould may lead one's life in an unpleasant, amputated or truncated condition which was not thought of.

In simple words, life is like a rainbow with varying colours which can be used to design and beautify our life with different combinations of attributes of our life.

LIFE FLOWS

At any moment, life continuously flows from a higher potential to a lower potential perpetually and is never static. The drive or impulse for different levels of potential is formed naturally or created artificially in different fields in the form of aim, encouragement, incentive, needs, enjoyment, etc.

The variety of attributes associated with life—mind, body, and the natural environment—is formed or appears to form a difference in potential naturally depending on the preference or taste of a person or a society. One may be hungry, another may be running after money, a third person may be running short of time to do his work and so on.

An artificially higher potential can be created by work in a field or in some fields sometimes. Since change in the potential is natural, keeping the level always high may not be possible. Hence, a person who never strives to achieve a higher level in a field is superseded by others in that field.

No person is complete at any time as far as the physical and psychological needs are concerned. Preferring the opposite gender, feeling superior because of the complexion of a person, feeling lonely, trying to do something which others find wonderful or difficult, trying to tell the ordeals or discoveries made in a journey, feeling awe struck by the enchanting colours of the dress of a person sitting nearby, etc. form a natural potential difference which cannot be stopped perpetually.

Life flows, both physically and psychologically.

SUPPLY AND DEMAND

The requirements and their availability at a reasonable cost or reasonable time or on our own terms always follow the natural law—when there is a need, the chances of getting it is less on our terms and conditions. In summer, the need for water is more, but the availability is less. In winter, the need for warmth is more, but the sun hardly helps in this respect.

The needs of a person make the life flow, and the toils of the person help to achieve them. But strangely enough, there is a time when everyone gets the demands fulfilled naturally, just like the seasonal flooding of goods and services. In an apple season or mango season, the abundance of these items enables everyone to get a share at a reasonable cost.

A person who desires to earn more money has to save when the supply is more and supply them when the demand is more. That is, one has to toil against the flow of nature. Similarly, a person who wants to lead a comfortable life has to save more money, an artificial storage of goods and services. A person who wants to enjoy life has to spend more money and time without worrying about the future. Thus, the supply and demand is rarely in equilibrium.

Strangely enough, the needs in life are more for sometimes continuously, and on some other time, one gets more than one needs continuously. It is the wise who saves when the supply is more and draws from the savings when the needs are more. A person who enjoys life when the supply is more finds life miserable when the demands in life are more. The ebb and flow in life last for some time, just like the seasons. That is, even though pain and pleasure in life are not permanent, pain or pleasure does not come or go in a flash.

Those who feel satisfied in life attain equilibrium and take rest till external or internal impulses push them to an active life.

Strangely enough, those who do not have, aspire while those who have, waste or misuse.

LIFE IN SIMILES AND METAPHORS

Many people are following the leader, just like sheep which follow the shepherd faithfully even though the shepherd will sell them to a butcher. There was a man who roared like a lion, and the whole crowd meekly accepted his proposal. Just like a mighty lion being challenged by a few hyenas, an honest leader is defeated by a coalition of a few unscrupulous people. This dame is as beautiful as a flower. He is a lion who defeated all his enemies single-handedly. That man is as loyal to his master as a dog.

Just like a bear which robs the hard-earned honey of the bees, a robber takes away the whole savings of a family. This man does all work at a snail's pace. This couple lives faithfully just like hawks in the wild. Just like a flock of deers fears on seeing a lion, all the villagers dispersed on seeing the local thug. Even though each one is fearful of the robber, all the villagers dared the robber, just like a herd of bisons drives away a lion. Without understanding, this boy recites the rhymes just like a parrot. This man enlightens the people who seek his advice, just like a tree which gives fruits to those who come near it. Just like a fish in the mouth of the shark, this man will be forced to give all his wealth to the moneylender. Just like a mosquito which lives on the blood of a person and, at the same time, spreads malaria, this man lives on the alms of society but humiliates and ill-treats the members of the society who gave alms. If a lion has its invisible boundary, then a dog has its own boundary. Similarly, this local thug's boundary covers the whole village.

Man being the last animal in the series of evolution, the characteristics of animals and other living things are enshrined in the hearts of humans at any time, and we do not know what is in the mind of a person at any moment—a hiding tiger or a fearing deer or something else.

EPIGRAPH

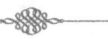

Live a full life, with effort to shape life according to one's perception within one's sphere of influence and with less emphasis on selfishness. A person with a conscience will feel the burden of responsibility.

We are paid back with the same coin-in the form of good wife or husband, understanding son or daughter, good health, reasonable intelligence, good patron, good friends, etc. —not necessarily in the form of money, power, etc. that we aspire to have.

But life flows so that a person enjoying the warmth under the sun may seek the darkness of night and a person wallowing in darkness may seek the light of day in the course of time.

Man and woman are shaped more by the society, family, and the knowledge and effort of the individuals than by the hereditary genes.

ENDNOTES

*   *Gargling*: It is used to clear a kind of throat infection which affects breathing seriously. Dissolve maximum possible amount of salt in a mouthful of warm water(NOT hot water) and pour it into your mouth. By keeping your face upward and taking deep breath, tell 'ha . . . ha . . ha...' for about a few seconds without swallowing the salt-water. After normal breathing for about 10 seconds, this can be repeated for a few minutes, preferably five minutes. After about five minutes, spit the salt water out and *clean your mouth with pure water to avoid any problem related to high blood pressure*. This kills some types of bacteria in the throat and some bacteria in the teeth and gums.

Throat infection seriously affects breathing and hence causes undiagnosable symptoms including regurgitation, inability to do any work, problem in sexual arousal for males, sudden and sharp pain in blood which comes and goes in a flash, etc. Gargling helps in proper breathing and mostly clears blocked nose. The major causes of throat infections are teeth infection, lung infection, inhalation through the mouth, eating spoiled food or spoiled fruits, or not cleaning the food particles in the mouth with water after eating or not brushing the teeth, particularly, in the night.

Some other kind of bacteria in the throat and respiratory tract can be killed by the hot air exhaled after doing heavy work like running, playing an outdoor game, etc. Gargling does not work for this kind of bacteria affecting the throat and respiratory tract, for which inhalation of steam from boiled water is needed. But never take hot food or hot drinks to soothe the throat. It may damage the teeth or the food pipe(oesophagus). Prefer warm food. Avoid hot dry air also to kill the bacteria.

** **Deep breathing exercise:** Standing up, take deep breath towards the forehead so that the chest and stomach expands, keep it for a few seconds or as long as you can hold your breath, and then exhale it slowly. Fast exhalation may cause headache. After each exercise, breath normally for about 10 seconds or more. Avoid doing this deep breathing exercise sitting down, since heart problems may arise. Prefer to do this deep breathing exercise for about 15 minutes in the morning and evening.

This deep breathing exercise causes the diaphragm, a muscular partition which separates the chest cavity and the abdominal cavity, to constrict and expand. It is rainbow shaped or dome shaped. The lungs expand when more air is inhaled and the diaphragm constricts and becomes flat. When the diaphragm expands and attains its dome-like curvature, the lungs constrict and exhale air. This expansion and constriction of diagram, due to deep breathing exercise, help both in digestion and in the smooth movement of the stools. So, constipation can be avoided by deep breathing exercise.

Since more oxygen(pure air) is absorbed in the blood through lungs, more sugar is burnt properly (just like a smokeless flame, and not like a wood burnt with less oxygen causing smoke.) for energy and work and so diabetes can be avoided. Due to proper pure blood flow to all organs, and timely removal of wastes from the body, high blood pressure can be avoided. Too much hard work, with less oxygen in the blood, produces more wastes in the body and so, it does not help to reduce blood sugar level.

Take deep breath towards the forehead so that the chest and stomach expand almost equally. Too much expansion of chest may reduce high blood pressure only marginally. Too much expansion of stomach may cause low blood pressure and men may experience problems of sexual erection. Keeping the stomach stiff for sometime may cause high blood pressure which normally occurs when one is in tension.

Sitting idly for long hours daily for years together affects breathing, which, in turn, affects blood flow to reproductive organs and hence women may face menstrual problems and men may face sexual erection problems. Most of the problems related to reproductive organs may be related to improper blood supply. Deep breathing exercise may mitigate the problems to some extent. Avoid continuous sitting for more than an hour at a time and stand up or walk for about five minutes after every hour.